TITLE: Skin Color and Health - Risks, Benefits, and Cultural Perspectives

Prologue: Imagine a journey through time, tracing the intricate threads of human evolution and adaptation. Picture a world where the sun's rays dance upon diverse skin hues, each shade a testament to survival, adaptation, and the relentless march of human progress. This book embarks on a journey through the evolutionary tale of human skin color, exploring how it shapes our health, history, cultural perspectives, and future developments in gene editing.

Unlock your skin's secrets with "Skin Color and Health: Risks, Benefits, and Cultural Perspectives." This comprehensive guide delves into the intricate relationship between skin color and health, offering invaluable insights for readers looking to understand skin's scientific, medical, and cultural aspects.

The book also sheds light on pigmentation's significant role in creating the vibrant colors and the rigidity of birds' feathers, a fascinating aspect of nature frequently overlooked in discussions about human pigmentation (Thompson, 2015).

Discover:

- **Health Benefits and Risks:** Learn how skin colors affect health, from UV protection and vitamin D synthesis to skin cancer risks and autoimmune diseases.

- **Genetic Foundations:** Explore the genetic basis of skin pigmentation and learn more about the intricacies of melanin production.

- **Treatment Strategies:** Get practical advice on managing skin-related health issues, including preventing vitamin D deficiency and skin cancer.

- **Cultural Perspectives:** Understand how skin color has shaped cultural identities and social dynamics throughout history and discover how stereotypes create barriers that prevent us from seeing each other as individuals and keep us from working together, hiring, or forming friendships.

- **Future Directions:** Stay informed about the latest advancements in genetic research and the potential of CRISPR technology in treating pigmentation disorders.

- **"Skin Color and Health - Risks, Benefits, and Cultural Perspectives"** is essential for anyone interested in dermatology (briefly), genetics, public health, or cultural studies. Whether you're a healthcare professional, a researcher, or simply curious about the science behind skin color, this book provides a well-rounded, accessible, and engaging exploration of one of the most conspicuous aspects of human diversity.

- **Skin Tanning** – Discover why skin tanning is bad for your health.

It also sheds light on pigmentation's significant role in creating the vibrant colors and rigidity of bird feathers, a fascinating aspect of nature often overlooked in discussions about human pigmentation (Thompson, 2015)

Introduction to Human Skin Color Evolution: As Jones sat by the window, watching the sun's rays play on the leaves of the old oak tree outside his school, he marvelled at how sunlight could warm your skin and create such vibrant life around you, and yet, is a gateway to a profound mystery that has shaped human history for millions of years. Human skin color, a trait as old as our species, has evolved in response to the sunlight that now bathed him in its gentle glow.

His understanding of human skin color, a multifaceted trait sculpted over millions of years by environmental forces such as UV radiation and climate, is crucial. The spectrum of skin colors we see today results from genetic adaptations that have enabled humans to flourish in various environments. By understanding the significance of human skin color, we can unravel the evolutionary origins of this trait, shedding light on the intricate whirl between our genes and the environments we inhabit. Recent genetic research has illuminated the underlying mechanisms of human skin pigmentation **(Jablonski and Chaplin, 2017).** This scientific exploration has not only deepened our understanding of human skin color but also provided valuable insights into the evolutionary journey of human populations and the genetic adaptations that have created the beautiful diversity of skin colors across the globe. It's a journey of enlightenment that we're excited to share with you.

Chapter 1: The Origins of Human Skin Color

Jones often wondered what life was like for the first humans. He might have imagined them walking under the blazing sun, their skin dark and resilient. It was a protective shield, nature's gift to help them survive the sun's harsh rays. As he pictured them migrating, their skin slowly adapting, lightening as they ventured into mild and less sunny climates, Jones realized that human skin color was a tale of survival and adaptation.

The Ancestral Skin Color of Early Humans

Scientists studying the evolution of human pigmentation are particularly interested in and debate the skin color of early humans. Modern humans display a wide range of skin tones. Our earliest ancestors were believed to have significantly darker skin, a crucial adaptation for survival in environments with intense sunlight (Jablonski and Chaplin, 2017).

Jones had just met up with Athenaca when the discussion about the history of skin color started.

Athenaca: Jones, as humans migrated from Africa to regions with less intense sunlight, their skin gradually lightened to allow for better vitamin D absorption, essential for bone health.

A complex interplay of genetics, environment, and cultural practices influences skin color. While the ancestral skin color of early humans may have been darker, modern skin tones result from genetic adaptations and environmental influences over tens of thousands of years. By studying the ancestral skin color of early humans, researchers aim to understand the evolutionary processes that have shaped the diversity of human skin tones seen today, illuminating our shared history as a species(Loomis, 1967).

The Role of UV Radiation in Evolution

Imagine the journey of early humans migrating out of Africa. Their skin color adapted as they moved into areas with varying UV radiation levels. In regions with intense sunlight, darker skin is protected against harmful UV rays, preventing skin cancer and folate depletion. In contrast, lighter skin evolved in some areas. Lower UV radiation enhances vitamin D synthesis, crucial for bone health and immune function.

Case Study: Indigenous Peoples of Australia:

The Aborigines

Background

Indigenous Australians, the Aborigines, one of the oldest continuous cultures on Earth, provide fascinating insights into human adaptation to diverse environments. Their skin color reflects a balance between UV protection and vitamin D synthesis in varying climates.

Genetic Makeup and Skin Color

Aborigines generally have darker skin, which is an adaptation to the high UV radiation in their environment. This pigmentation protects against UV damage, reducing the risk of skin cancer while maintaining adequate vitamin D levels through dietary sources like fish and other seafood.

Cultural Practices and Health

The Aborigines have rich cultural practices, including traditional fishing and hunting techniques that provide vitamin D-rich foods. These practices and their genetic adaptations have helped them thrive in their environment for thousands of years.

Evolutionary Mechanisms

Genetic Variants and Skin Color:

The genetic basis of skin color involves several essential genes, including MC1R, SLC24A5, and TYR. Variations in these genes influence melanin production and distribution, leading to diverse skin colors. For instance, MC1R variants are associated with red hair and fair skin, while SLC24A5 variants are linked to lighter skin tones in European populations.

Evolutionary Pressure:

Natural selection has played a crucial role in shaping skin color. In high UV regions, darker skin was favored for its protective properties. In contrast, lighter skin evolved in areas with lower UV radiation to enhance vitamin D synthesis. This balance between protection and vitamin D production highlights the adaptive nature of human skin color.

Case Study: The Maasai of East Africa

Background

The Maasai people of East Africa are renowned for their vibrant culture and unique adaptations to their environment. Living in regions with intense sunlight, their skin color reflects evolutionary adaptations to high UV radiation.

Genetic Makeup and Skin Color

The Maasai have relatively dark skin, protecting against UV radiation. This adaptation is crucial for preventing skin cancer and maintaining folate levels. Despite high UV exposure, the Maasai maintain adequate vitamin D levels through a diet rich in vitamin D sources like milk and blood from cattle.

Cultural Practices and Health

The Maasai's pastoral lifestyle involves spending significant time outdoors, necessitating their dark skin for UV protection. Their diet, rich in vitamin D, complements their genetic adaptations, ensuring overall health and resilience in their environment.

Case Study: The Khoisan of Southern Africa

Background: The Khoisan people, comprising the San (Bushmen) and Khoikhoi (Hottentots), are Indigenous to Southern Africa and possess a unique genetic makeup. As one of the oldest genetic lineages, the Khoisan provides critical insights into early human evolution(Wikipedia, 2024).

Genetic Makeup and Skin Color

The Khoisan have a relatively light skin tone compared to other African populations living closer to the equator. This adaptation is linked to their environment, which has lower UV radiation levels. Their skin color results from genetic variations that evolved over thousands of years to balance UV protection with adequate vitamin D synthesis.

"Imagine," said Jones, "living in the semi-arid regions of the Kalahari Desert with their unique body structure."

"Exactly," Athenaca continued. "They have shorter statures and long limbs, which help in thermoregulation."

Adaptations and Survival

Living in the semi-arid regions of the Kalahari Desert, the Khoisan have developed several adaptations to survive their harsh environment. These include:

- **Melanin Levels:** While they have lighter skin than equatorial Africans, the Khoisan still possess enough melanin to protect against UV radiation in their environment. This balance between UV protection and sufficient vitamin D production is a testament to their adaptation.
- **Body Structure:** The Khoisan have a unique body structure with a relatively short stature and long limbs, aiding in thermoregulation. This adaptation allows them to dissipate heat more effectively in the hot, dry climate of the Kalahari Desert.
- **Diet and Nutrition:** Traditionally, the Khoisan diet consists of plant-based foods rich in nutrients and proteins from hunting small game. This diet provides the necessary vitamins and minerals to support their health in a challenging environment.

Cultural Practices and Health

The Khoisan have a rich cultural heritage with practices that have evolved to suit their environment. These include:

- **Traditional Healing:** The Khoisan use various medicinal plants for healing purposes. Their extensive knowledge of local flora and its medicinal properties is passed down through generations.

- **Social Structure:** The Khoisan society is egalitarian, with decisions made through consensus. This social structure promotes cooperation and resource sharing,

which are crucial for survival in a harsh environment.

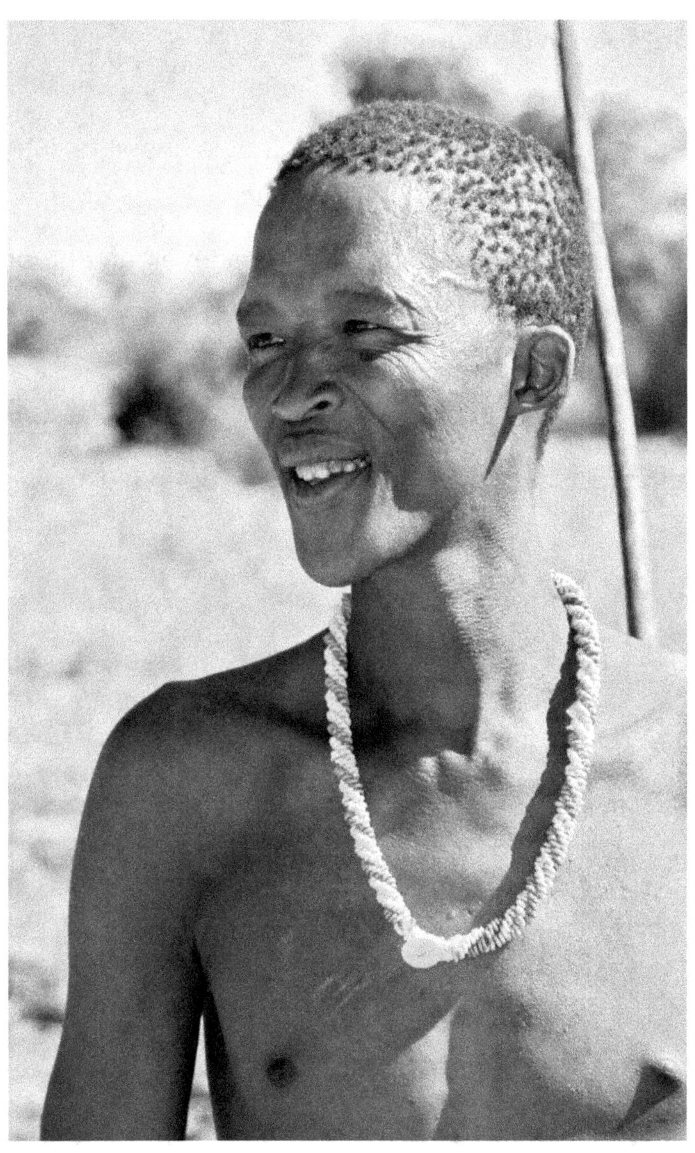

Figure 1 - A Khoisan of South Africa - Taken from:(Wikipedia, 2024).

Implications for Modern Research

Studies of the Khoisan people provide valuable insights into human adaptation and evolution. Their genetic makeup offers clues about early human migrations and the development of genetic traits that allowed humans to survive in diverse environments. Understanding these adaptations helps researchers appreciate the complexity of human evolution and the role of genetic diversity in our survival(Wikipedia, 2024).

Case Study: The Inuit of the Arctic

Background

The Inuit people, indigenous to the Arctic regions of Canada, Greenland, and Alaska, have adapted to one of the harshest climates on Earth. Their environment is characterized by extreme cold, low sunlight, and a diet heavily dependent on marine resources.

Genetic Makeup and Skin Color: Despite living in high latitudes with limited sunlight, the Inuit have a darker skin tone than other populations at similar latitudes. This is believed to be an adaptation linked to their traditional diet, which is rich in vitamin D from marine mammals like seals and whales.

"Jones," said Athenaca with a focused expression, "do you know why the Inuit have darker skin despite living in low UV regions?"

Jones shrugged. "Their diet?"

"Exactly," **Athenaca replied.** "Their diet is high in vitamin D, so they don't need to synthesize as much from sunlight."

Adaptations and Survival

The Inuit have developed numerous adaptations to thrive in the Arctic environment:

- **Skin Color and Vitamin D:** The Inuit diet, high in vitamin D, reduces the evolutionary pressure for lighter skin to synthesize vitamin D from sunlight. This dietary adaptation allows them to maintain a darker skin tone, providing some protection against the intense reflection of UV rays from snow and ice.
- **Body Structure:** The Inuit have a compact body structure with a higher percentage of body fat, which helps them insulate against the cold. Their short, stocky build minimizes heat loss and conserves energy in the frigid climate.
- **Metabolism:** The Inuit have a unique metabolic adaptation that allows them to process fatty acids from their marine-based diet efficiently. This adaptation is crucial for maintaining energy levels and overall health in a low-carbohydrate environment.

Cultural Practices and Health:

The Inuit culture is rich in traditions that support their survival in the Arctic:

- **Hunting and Gathering:** The Inuit are skilled hunters, relying on techniques passed down through generations to hunt seals, whales, and fish. These practices ensure a steady supply of food rich in essential nutrients.
- **Clothing and Shelter:** Traditional Inuit clothing, made from animal skins and furs, provides excellent insulation against the cold. Igloos and other traditional shelters are designed to retain heat and protect against harsh weather conditions
- **Community and Social Structure:** Inuit society is close-knit, with strong family ties and communal living. This social structure promotes sharing resources and mutual support, which is essential for survival in a challenging environment.

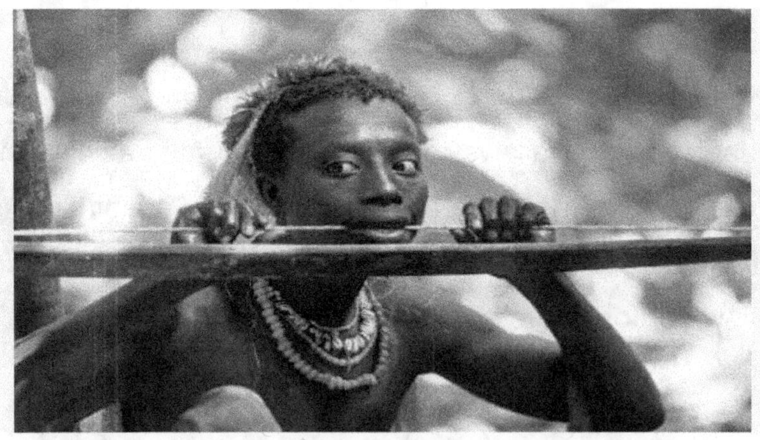

Figure 2 - Showing an Inuit of the Arctic

Implications for Modern Research

The Inuit people offer a unique perspective on human adaptation to extreme environments. Their genetic and cultural adaptations provide valuable insights into how humans can thrive in diverse and challenging climates. Studying the Inuit helps researchers understand the interplay between genetics, diet, and environment in shaping human health and survival.

Narrative: A Dermatologist's Perspective: **Dr Susan Taylor's Insights:** Dr Susan Taylor, a renowned dermatologist specializing in the skin of color, shares her experiences and insights into the prevalence of skin conditions among different skin tones. Her practice addresses the unique challenges faced by individuals with darker skin, who often experience different dermatological issues compared to those with lighter skin.

Common Skin Conditions: Dr Taylor discusses several skin conditions prevalent among people with darker skin tones:

- **Hyperpigmentation**: This condition, characterized by dark patches on the skin, is more common in individuals with darker skin. It often results from inflammation, injury, or acne and can be challenging to treat.
- **Keloids**: People with darker skin are more prone to developing keloids, which are raised scars that grow excessively at the site of a skin injury. Treating keloids

requires specialized techniques to minimize their appearance and prevent recurrence.

- **Vitiligo**: This condition causes depigmented patches and can be particularly distressing for individuals with darker skin. Dr Taylor emphasizes the importance of
- tailored treatment plans that address vitiligo's medical and psychological aspects.
- **Freckles:** Freckles are a type of hyperpigmentation. People with them produce more than enough melanin but does not distribute evenly across the skin. This causes the little localised areas of discolouration, fondly (or not!) known as freckles.

Treatment of freckles: Chemical Peels:

- **Peeling Agents:** Chemical peels using agents like trichloroacetic acid (TCA) or glycolic acid can help exfoliate the skin, reduce pigmentation, and improve the overall appearance of freckles

Natural Remedies:

- **Lemon Juice:** Lemon juice is a natural bleaching agent and can help lighten freckles over time. However, it should be used cautiously, as it can make the skin more sensitive to sunlight.
- **Honey and Buttermilk:** These natural ingredients have mild bleaching properties and can be used as a mask to reduce the appearance of freckles.

- **Intense Pulsed Light (IPL):** IPL is a non-invasive treatment that uses light energy to target pigmented cells, reducing the appearance of freckles over multiple sessions.

Treatment Approaches

Dr Taylor highlights the importance of personalized treatment approaches for patients with different skin tones:

- **Topical Treatments**: She recommends using specific formulations of topical treatments that are effective and safe for darker skin. These include hydroquinone for hyperpigmentation and silicone gel sheets for keloid management.
- **Laser Therapy:** Dr Taylor explains that laser therapy can be effective for certain conditions but requires careful selection of the type of laser and settings to avoid
- complications like hyperpigmentation or hypopigmentation in darker skin.
- **Patient Education:** It is crucial to educate patients about their skin type and the appropriate care. Dr. Taylor emphasizes the importance of sun protection and sunscreen, even for individuals with darker skin, to prevent further pigmentation issues and skin cancer.

SKIN cancer – tanning - Exposure to ultraviolet (UV) radiation can lead to damage to your skin and eyes, as well as elevate the risk of developing skin cancer. If you observe your skin beginning to change color, often referred to as a 'tan,' it indicates that your body is attempting to shield itself from UV radiation. Tanning beds or sunbeds do not offer a safe way to achieve a tan. While fake tanning lotions might be a safer alternative for altering skin tone, they typically do not protect against the sun.

How Skin Tans— In the simplest terms, tanning is the darkening of the skin due to exposure to ultraviolet (UV) light. When UV radiation reaches your skin, your body recognizes it as an injury and triggers chemical changes in specific skin cells. To protect itself, your skin darkens to block harmful rays and prevent further damage. A more profound tan results from the darkening of existing pigment and a slight increase in new pigment production(*Section One- What Causes Tanning Of The Skin? | Utah County Health Department*, no date).

There is no such thing as a 'safe' suntan. Any method that exposes your skin to UV radiation will result in skin damage. The more your skin is exposed to UV radiation, the higher your risk of developing skin cancer, and the faster your skin will age.(*Skin cancer - tanning - Better Health Channel*, no date).

Dr Taylor's Impact: Dr Taylor's contributions to dermatology for skin color have been significant. Her research and clinical practice have improved the understanding and treatment of skin conditions in diverse populations. Her advocacy for patient education and personalized care continues to impact the field positively. Dr Taylor has spearheaded numerous initiatives promoting skin-of-color dermatology at the University of Pennsylvania and for dermatology nationwide. She founded the Skin of Color Centre at St. Luke's Roosevelt Hospital in New York City and the Skin of Color Society, which promotes awareness and excellence in skin of color dermatology.

Narrative: A Geneticist's Journey: Dr Sarah Tishkoff's Research: Dr Sarah Tishkoff, a leading geneticist, has extensively studied African populations to understand the genetic basis of skin color. Her research has uncovered important insights into how genetic variations contribute to the diversity of human skin tones.

Fundamental Discoveries: Dr Tishkoff's research has led to several ground-breaking discoveries:

- **Genetic Variants**: She has identified numerous genetic variants associated with skin pigmentation in African populations. These variants help explain the wide range of skin colors observed within and between different populations.
- **Evolutionary History**: Her work has revealed the evolutionary history of these genetic variants, showing how natural selection has shaped skin color adaptations in response to varying environmental pressures.

- **Health Implications**: Dr Tishkoff's research has also explored the health implications of these genetic
- variations. For example, specific variants associated with darker skin protect against UV damage but may also influence other health outcomes, such as susceptibility to certain skin conditions.

Research Challenges: Dr Tishkoff shares the challenges she has faced in her research journey:

- **Fieldwork in Africa**: Conducting genetic research in diverse African populations requires extensive fieldwork, often in remote areas. Dr Tishkoff's dedication to building relationships with local communities and ensuring ethical research practices has been essential to her success.
- **Data Analysis**: Analysing genetic data from diverse populations presents unique challenges due to the high genetic diversity and complex population histories. Dr Tishkoff's innovative analytical approaches have been crucial in overcoming these challenges.
- **Collaborative Efforts**: Her research has involved collaboration with scientists from various disciplines, including anthropology, biology, and medicine. These interdisciplinary efforts have enriched her understanding of the genetic and environmental factors influencing skin color.

Personal Reflections: Dr Tishkoff reflects on the personal impact of her research:

- NSF Sloan Postdoctoral fellowship in molecular evolution, 1996-1998

David and Lucile Packard Career Award in Science and Engineering, 2001-2006

NIH Pioneer Award, 2009

- **Educational Mission**: Dr Tishkoff is committed to educating the public and the scientific community about the complexities of human genetic diversity. She advocates for more excellent representation of diverse populations in genetic research to ensure that the benefits of scientific discoveries are shared equitably.

Awards: NSF Sloan Postdoctoral fellowship in molecular evolution, 1996-1998, David and Lucile Packard Career Award in Science and Engineering, 2001-2006, NIH Pioneer Award, 2009.

Dr Tishkoff's Legacy: Dr Tishkoff's contributions to genetic research have significantly advanced our understanding of human skin color. Her work has highlighted the importance of studying diverse populations to uncover the full spectrum of human genetic diversity. Her commitment to ethical research practices and public education continues to inspire future generations of scientists.

She has conducted combined fieldwork, laboratory experiments, and computational methods to explore key questions about modern human evolutionary history and the genetic structure of traits linked to adaptation and disease risk in Africa. Using an integrative genomics approach, Their research incorporates genomic, proteomic, epigenetic, transcriptomic, metabolomic, and microbiome data from ethnically diverse African populations living in various environments to identify genetic and environmental factors influencing a range of anthropometric, metabolomic, cardiovascular, and immune-related traits**(Tishkoff Lab / Sarah Tishkoff, Ph.D., no date).**

The Role of Pigmentation in the Creation of the Colorful Feathers of Birds: One afternoon, Jones sat under the sprawling oak tree, flipping through the pages of his biology textbook. The summer sun filtered through the leaves, casting dappled shadows on the grass. He looked up as Athenaca approached, her presence always accompanied by a sense of calm wisdom.

"Athenaca," Jones began, his brow furrowed with curiosity. Pigmentation also plays a part in the colors and structure of birds' feathers. I've been reading about how these colors are formed. It's fascinating but a bit complex. Could you help me understand it better?"

Athenaca smiled, settling down beside him. "Of course, Jones. Birds, indeed, have a remarkable way of creating their colorful feathers. They use two main mechanisms: pigmentation and structural colors. Let's start with pigmentation."

"Pigments, right," Jones nodded, "but what kinds specifically?"

"Three primary pigments contribute to bird coloration," Athenaca explained. "First, there are carotenoids. These are pigments that birds acquire through their diet. Carotenoids produce bright reds, yellows, and oranges. Imagine the vibrant hues of the Northern Cardinal or the Blackburnian Warbler."(Thompson, 2015).

"So, their diet directly influences their feather colors?" Jones asked.

"Exactly," Athenaca confirmed. "Then, we have melanins. These pigments are found in both the skin and feathers of birds. They provide a range of colors from black to reddish-brown and yellow. But melanins do more than just color feathers—they also strengthen them. Melanin-rich feathers are more resistant to wear and tear."(Thompson, 2015).

Jones scribbled notes in his book, glancing up with a question in his eyes. "And what about porphyrins? I've read they have something to do with UV light."

Athenaca nodded. "Porphyrins are indeed fascinating. These pigments fluoresce under UV light, creating vivid greens and reds. You can see this in birds like the turacos. It's a brilliant example of nature's ingenuity."(Thompson, 2015).

Jones leaned back, taking in the information. "So, pigments handle many of the colors, but what about those shimmering, changing colors you see in some birds?"

"That's where structural colors come into play," Athenaca said, her eyes lighting up enthusiastically. "Structural colors are created by the microscopic structure of the feathers rather than pigments. For example, iridescent (sparkling) feathers cause light to refract through their microstructures. This creates colors that change with the viewing angle. Hummingbirds and the Purple Gallinule are perfect examples."(Thompson, 2015).

Jones's eyes widened. "And non-iridescent feathers? How do they work?"

"Non-iridescent structural colors are produced by light scattering from air pockets in the feather barbs," Athenaca explained. "This scattering effect can create colors like blue. Looking at a Blue Jay or a bluebird in backlighting, the feathers appear brown due to the underlying melanin layer. It's a beautiful interplay of light and structure."(Thompson, 2015

Jones looked thoughtful. "So, the colors we see combine pigments and structural features?"

"Precisely," Athenaca said, smiling. "It's a complex interplay that results in the stunning array of visual effects we see in bird feathers. Sometimes, birds can exhibit color abnormalities due to unusual levels of pigments. For instance, partial albinism can occur in species like American Crows and Canada Geese, leading to unique color changes."

Jones closed his textbook, a newfound appreciation for the subject in his eyes. "Thanks, Athenaca. This makes so much more sense now. Nature's complexity never ceases to amaze me."

Athenaca nodded, her gaze drifting to the sky where a cardinal flashed its bright red wings. "Indeed, Jones. The more we learn, the more we realize there's always more to discover. (Thompson, 2015)

Carotenoids

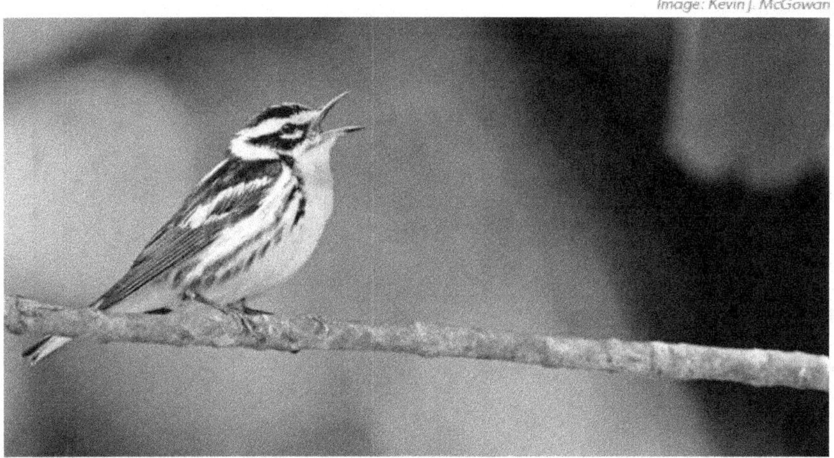

Male Blackburnian Warbler throat and chest feathers contain carotenoid pigments

Figure 3 - Showing A Male Blackburnian Warbler displaying the yellow color from carotenoid pigments. (Thompson, 2015).

Melanins

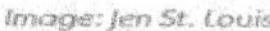

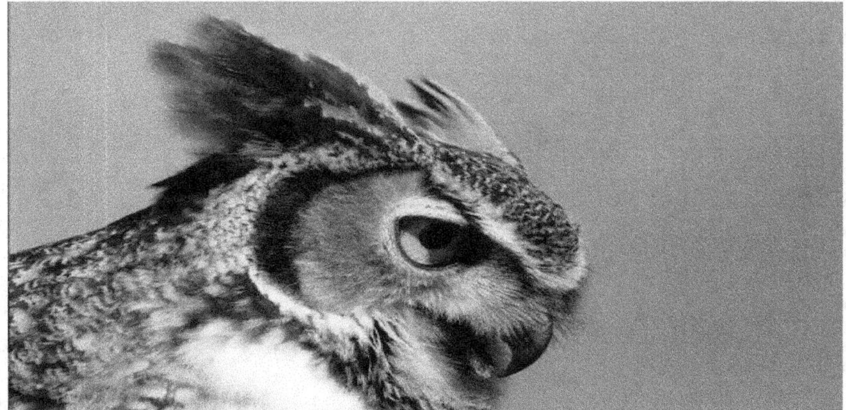

Great Horned Owl feathers contain melanin pigment

Figure 4 - Showing an Owl with feathers containing melanin pigment(Thompson, 2015).

Porphyrins

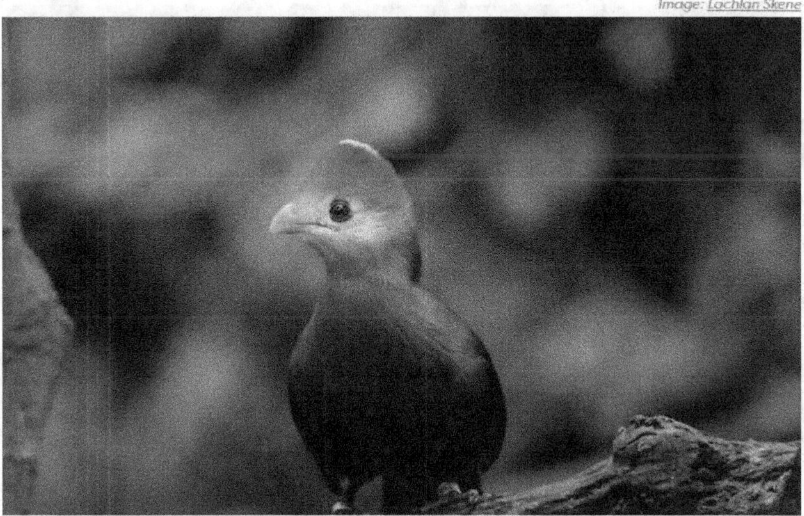

Red-crested Turaco feathers contain pigments derived from porphyrins

Figure 5 - Showing Red-created Turaco feathers containing pigment obtained from porphyrins(Thompson, 2015).

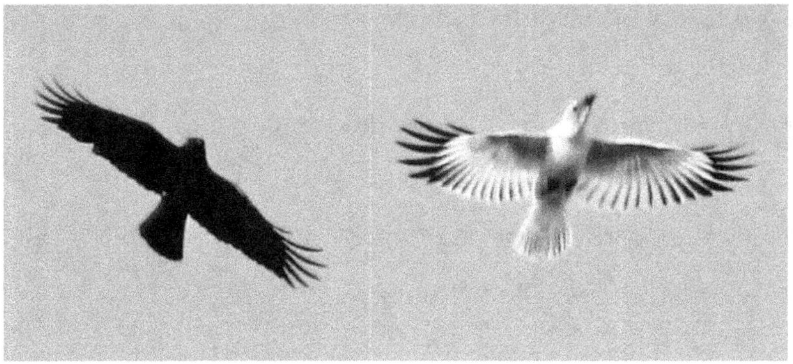

Two American Crows, the bird on the right has lower than normal levels of melanin pigments:

Figure 6 - Showing two crows, with the crow on the right displaying lower than normal levels of melanin pigments(Thompson, 2015)

Chapter 2: Production and Protective Roles Against UV Radiation

One sunny afternoon, Jones lay on the grass, contemplating the sun's invisible rays that warmed his skin. He pondered how something unseen could profoundly affect his body, protecting it yet potentially harming it. This curious dance between the sun and our skin has fascinated scientists for centuries, leading to the discovery of melanin, the guardian of our skin.

What is Melanin?

The origin of the term melanin, from the Greek word melanos("dark" or "black"), is frequently attributed to the Swedish chemist Berzelius(Fedorow and Double, 2005). Based on their precursor molecules, melanins are classified into four groups(Fedorow and Double, 2005):

Eumelanin is formed from l-3,4-dihydroxyphenylalanine (l-dopa).

Pheomelanin is formed by oxidative polymerization of 5-*S*-cysteinyl-dopa or 2-*S*-cysteinyl-dopa.

Neuromelanin is thought to be formed by oxidative polymerization of dopamine or noradrenaline, possibly involving cysteinyl-derivatives.

Allomelanin is formed by the oxidation of polyphenols, such as catechols and 1,8-dihydroxynaphtalene. They are widely spread in fungi and are often nitrogen-free.

Melanin is a pigment that determines the color of our skin, hair, and eyes. It is produced by cells called melanocytes. Our genetics influence the amount and type of melanin produced, although factors such as exposure to sunlight can also affect its production. Melanin plays a crucial role in protecting our skin from the harmful effects of UV radiation, which can cause skin cancer and premature aging(Jablonski and Chaplin, 2017).

Jones sat cross-legged on a large cushion in the study, surrounded by towering bookshelves filled with ancient tomes and scientific journals. His mentor, Athenaca, paced slowly by the window, her thoughtful gaze lost in the play of sunlight filtering through the leaves outside.

"Athenaca," Jones began, "I've been reading about the role of melanin in our skin and how it affects vitamin D production. It's fascinating how something as simple as a pigment can significantly affect our health."

Athenaca turned to face him, her expression encouraging. "Indeed, Jones. Melanin, the pigment responsible for our skin color, is remarkable. It provides a natural sunscreen effect by absorbing UVB radiation."

"But," Jones interjected, "this protective quality of melanin also reduces the amount of UVB radiation available for synthesizing vitamin D, doesn't it?"

"Precisely," Athenaca said, nodding. "While melanin's ability to absorb UVB radiation protects us from sunburn and reduces the risk of skin cancer, it also means that individuals with darker skin tones, which contain more melanin, need more sun exposure to produce the same amount of vitamin D as those with lighter skin."

Jones's brow furrowed in thought. "How much more sun exposure are we talking about?"

"Research suggests," Athenaca explained, "that darker skin may require up to six times more sun exposure to produce the same amount of vitamin D as someone with lighter skin. This increased requirement puts people with darker skin at a higher risk of vitamin D deficiency."(Vitamin D Deficiency & Skin Type: What You Need to Know | Cue, 2023)

"That's quite significant," Jones mused. "The American Osteopathic Association has detailed studies on this topic, right?"

"Yes," Athenaca confirmed. "According to the National Institutes of Health, individuals with darker skin are more likely to have lower vitamin D levels. This deficiency can lead to symptoms like fatigue, muscle weakness, bone pain, and an increased risk of infections."(Vitamin D Deficiency & Skin Type: What You Need to Know | Cue, 2023)

Jones nodded, absorbing the information. "But these symptoms can be subtle and easily overlooked, can't they? It makes sense that people with darker skin need to be especially proactive about monitoring their vitamin D levels."(Vitamin D Deficiency & Skin Type: What You Need to Know | Cue, 2023)

"Exactly," Athenaca agreed. "Ethnicity also plays a role. African Americans, Hispanics, and South Asians are at greater risk of lower vitamin D levels compared to Caucasians due to differences in skin pigmentation. The Journal of the American Academy of Dermatology comprehensively reviews this subject."(Vitamin D Deficiency & Skin Type: What You Need to Know | Cue, 2023)

Jones leaned back, contemplating. "And what about those with fair skin? How does their melanin content affect their vitamin D production and overall health?"

"Individuals with lighter skin tones have less melanin, which allows them to absorb UVB radiation more efficiently," Athenaca explained. "This means they can produce vitamin D more effectively, but it also increases their risk of sunburn and skin cancer if they don't take proper sun protection measures."(Vitamin D Deficiency & Skin Type: What You Need to Know | Cue, 2023)

"So, while fair-skinned individuals are generally less likely to develop vitamin D deficiency, they aren't completely immune, especially if they live in areas with limited sunlight or have lifestyles that limit sun exposure," Jones concluded.

"Precisely," Athenaca affirmed. "It's essential for everyone, regardless of skin tone, to be aware of vitamin D deficiency symptoms. This can include mood changes, hair loss, and a weakened immune system for fair-skinned individuals."

Jones looked out the window, the sunlight dancing on his face. "It's incredible how something as seemingly simple as sunlight can have such complex and varied effects on our bodies."

Athenaca smiled with pride. "That's the beauty of learning, Jones. Every new piece of knowledge opens a world of understanding and awareness. And it's through these understandings that we can better care for ourselves and each other."

Types of Melanin, Their Functions & Production Types of Melanin and Their Functions:

There are two main types of melanin: eumelanin and pheomelanin. Eumelanin produces brown and black hues, while pheomelanin creates red and yellow tones. These two types of melanin work together to determine our overall skin color.

"Jones," Athenaca said, twirling a leaf between her fingers, "do you know the two types of melanin?"

"Eumelanin and pheomelanin," Jones replied, feeling like he was in a biology class.

"Correct," Athenaca smiled. "Eumelanin is like a natural sunscreen. More eumelanin means better protection from UV rays."

- **Eumelanin is the** most common type of melanin found in humans. It is a natural sunscreen that protects the skin from harmful UV rays. People with higher levels of eumelanin are less likely to suffer from sunburns and skin cancer. This explains why individuals with darker skin tones are better adapted to living in regions with intense sunlight**(Jablonski and Chaplin, 2017).**
- **Pheomelanin:** It is less effective at blocking UV rays and does not provide as much protection against sun damage. People with fair skin and red hair have higher levels of pheomelanin, making them more susceptible to sunburns

and skin cancer. Despite this disadvantage, pheomelanin also plays a role in creating unique hair and eye colors.

Genetic and evolutionary factors affect the distribution of eumelanin and pheomelanin in the skin.

As people migrated to different parts of the world, their skin color adapted to the local climate and sunlight exposure. This explains why populations living near the equator tend to have darker skin while those in higher latitudes have lighter skin. These adaptations helped early humans survive and thrive in their respective environments (Jablonski and Chaplin, 2017).

Genetic Influence

Genetic factors determine the amount and type of melanin produced by melanocytes. Variations in specific genes can influence the activity of enzymes and proteins in melanin synthesis, resulting in different skin pigmentation.

Jones: Hi, Athena. I still don't fully understand melanin production in the body, and I need some help understanding a few things about genetics for my biology class. Can you explain what the genes MC1R and SLC24A5 do? And what does the word "variant" mean in this context?

Athenaca: Of course, Jones! Let's break it down step by step. First, let's talk about the term "variant." In biology, a variant refers to a change or alteration in a gene's most common DNA nucleotide sequence. Think of it like a slight tweak in the genetic code.

Jones: A variant is a slight change in the gene's DNA sequence. I understand. Now, what about the MC1R gene?

Athenaca: The MC1R gene, which stands for Melanocortin 1 Receptor, is critical in determining hair and skin color. Typically, the MC1R gene produces a type of melanin called eumelanin, which gives us darker hair and skin tones**(MedlinePlus, 2024).**

Jones: So, does it make the darker pigment?

Athenaca: Exactly. However, variants in the MC1R gene can reduce the gene's activity. This reduced activity favors the production of another type of melanin called pheomelanin, which is associated with red hair and fair skin. People with these variants also tend to have increased sensitivity to UV radiation**(MedlinePlus, 2024).**

Jones: That makes sense! So, redheads with fair skin often have these variants in the MC1R gene?

Athenaca: Right! Now, let's move on to the SLC24A5 gene. This gene is part of the solute carrier family and regulates the amount of potassium and calcium in melanocytes, which produce melanin.

Jones: What does it do precisely with melanin production?

Athenaca: Variants in the SLC24A5 gene can affect melanin production, particularly eumelanin production. These variants are linked to lighter skin tones, especially in European populations. By reducing eumelanin production, these variants contribute to lighter skin**(MedlinePlus, 2024).**

Jones: So, the SLC24A5 gene variants are another reason some people have lighter skin?

Athenaca: Yes, that's correct. Both MC1R and SLC24A5 genes, through their variants, influence the type and amount of melanin produced, affecting hair and skin**(MedlinePlus, 2024).**

Jones: Thanks, Athenaca! This helps clarify how these genes and their variants work.

Athenaca: You're welcome, Jones! Genetics can seem complex, but breaking it down into simple terms makes it much easier to understand. Keep up the excellent work!

"To understand the production of melanin in the body, think of it like a factory," Athenaca explained. Genetic instructions are the blueprints, and the production lines create eumelanin or pheomelanin based on those instructions.

Think of melanin production as a factory where the genetic instructions act like blueprints. In this factory:

- **Tyrosinase:** This enzyme (An enzyme is a particular protein in our bodies that speeds up chemical reactions. Think of it like a helper that makes things happen faster and more efficiently) is the machinery that starts the production process, converting tyrosine into the initial product, dopaquinone.
- **Eumelanin Line:** If the factory receives instructions from genes like MC1R to produce more eumelanin, it will process dopaquinone through a series of steps to make brown or black eumelanin. This is akin to a production line creating durable, UV-resistant materials.
- **Pheomelanin Line:** If the instructions favor pheomelanin (due to genetic variations like those in MC1R), the factory diverts dopaquinone to produce red or yellow pheomelanin, like producing less UV-resistant materials.

Quality Control: Genetic variations can affect the efficiency and output of these production lines, resulting in the diverse range of skin colors observed in humans.

Detailed Mechanisms of Melanin Production

The Melanin Production Pathway

Melanin synthesis begins in melanocytes, where the enzyme tyrosinase converts the amino acid tyrosine into dopaquinone. This intermediate then follows one of two pathways to produce either eumelanin or pheomelanin. The balance between these two types of melanin determines overall skin color.

Role of Genetic Factors: Genetic factors are crucial in melanin production. Variants in the TYR gene, which encodes tyrosinase, can affect the enzyme's activity, leading to variations in melanin levels. Other genes, like OCA2, influence the transport and storage of melanin within melanocytes.

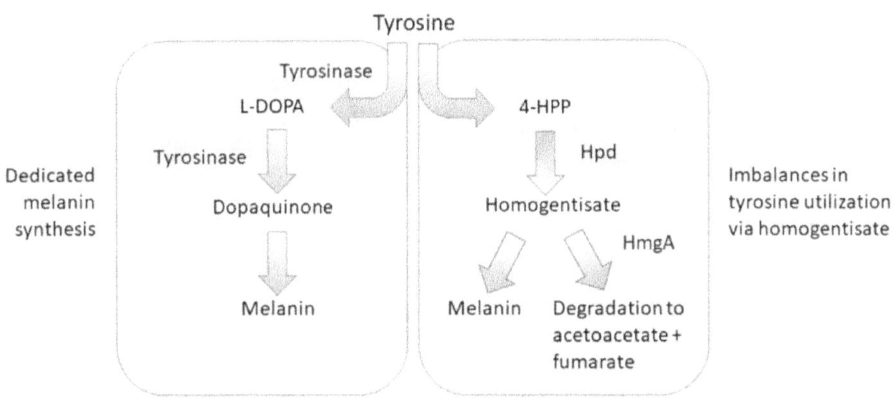

Simplified pathways of tyrosine-derived melanin synthesis showing enzymatic steps subject to regulation. L-DOPA, L-3,4-dihydroxyphenylalanine; 4-HPP, 4-hydroxyphenylpyruvate; Hpd, 4-hydroxyphenylpyruvate dioxygenase; HmgA, homogentisate 1,2-dioxygenase(Pavan, Lopez and Pettinari, 2020).

The tyrosinase MelC2 remains inactive until it is secreted and activated by MelC1 (chaperone for secretion and copper incorporation into the active site of MelC2). After the transportation, MelC1 dissociates from MelC2, which activates tyrosinase activity(Pavan, Lopez and Pettinari, 2020)

Health Implications of Melanin - Protection Against UV Radiation: Eumelanin effectively protects against UV-induced skin damage with its high UV-absorbing capacity. This protection reduces the risk of skin cancer and photoaging, making eumelanin-rich skin advantageous in high UV environments.

Vitamin D Synthesis and Bone Health

While melanin offers protection, it also limits UVB radiation absorption necessary for vitamin D synthesis. This trade-off highlights the evolutionary balance between protecting against UV damage and maintaining adequate vitamin D levels for bone health.

Case Study: Albinism and Its Implications

Background

Albinism is a genetic condition characterized by a lack of melanin production. It affects individuals worldwide and leads to significant health challenges.

Genetic Basis

Albinism results from mutations in genes involved in melanin production, such as TYR, OCA2, and SLC45A2. These mutations disrupt the melanin synthesis pathway, leading to reduced or absent melanin.

Health Implications: Individuals with albinism have very light skin and are highly susceptible to UV damage, increasing the risk of skin cancer. They also face vision-related challenges, as melanin plays a role in eye development. Addressing these health issues requires careful sun protection and regular medical check-ups.

By understanding the production and roles of eumelanin and pheomelanin, along with the genetic factors influencing their levels, we gain insights into the evolutionary adaptations of skin color and the health implications of UV radiation exposure.

Key Genes:

- **MC1R (Melanocortin 1 Receptor):** Variants (caused by alteration in the most common DNA nucleotide sequence**).** Alternatives to the MC1R gene can reduce the receptor's activity, favoring the production of pheomelanin over eumelanin. These variants are commonly associated with red hair, fair skin, and increased sensitivity to UV radiation**(MedlinePlus, 2024).**
- **SLC24A5 (Solute Carrier Family 24 Member 5):** This gene influences melanin production by regulating the amount of potassium and calcium in melanocytes. Variants of SLC24A5 are linked to lighter skin tones, particularly in European populations, by reducing eumelanin production**(MedlinePlus, 2024).**

Chapter 3: Migration and Skin Color Variation

Human Migration Patterns:

Jones: "Athenaca, I've been thinking a lot about how human migration has influenced our skin color. It's fascinating how our ancestors' movements shaped the diversity we see today."

Athenaca: "Indeed, Jones. Our journey from Africa to various parts of the world has profoundly impacted our biology, especially our skin color. It's a vivid illustration of how humans adapt to their environments."

Jones: "Right, so when our ancestors moved out of Africa, they encountered different climates and levels of UV radiation. Over time, their skin color evolved to suit these new conditions."

Athenaca: "Exactly. This process is known as natural selection. For instance, populations that stayed near the equator, where UV radiation is intense, developed darker skin. This high melanin content in their skin protects against the harmful effects of UV rays."

Jones: "Conversely, those who migrated to areas with less sunlight, like northern Europe, evolved to have lighter skin. This helped them absorb more UV radiation to produce vitamin D essential for bone health."

Athenaca: "Precisely. The need for vitamin D production was a significant selective pressure in higher latitudes. Lighter skin became advantageous in those regions because it allowed for better absorption of the limited sunlight available."

Jones: "Skin color is a clear example of how humans have adapted to their environments over millennia. It's about sun protection and other factors like temperature regulation."

Athenaca: "Yes, skin color adaptations are multifaceted. In hotter climates, darker skin can help dissipate heat more effectively.

Conversely, in colder regions, lighter skin may help retain heat. These adaptations have enabled humans to thrive in diverse environments."

Jones: "It's also intriguing how multiple genes, not just one, influence these changes. This explains the variety of skin tones we see among different populations."

Athenaca: "Absolutely. Our genetic makeup is incredibly complex, and the variation in skin color is a testament to that complexity. Each population's unique genetic heritage reflects its evolutionary history and environmental adaptations."

Jones: "Understanding this helps us appreciate our shared history as a species. Despite our differences in skin color, we're all interconnected and part of the same evolutionary journey."

Athenaca: "That's a crucial point, Jones. By studying human migration patterns and the evolution of skin color, we gain insights into our past and a deeper appreciation for the diversity and unity of the human species."

Jones: "It's amazing how science can reveal the stories written in our genes. It makes me wonder what other secrets our DNA holds about our ancestors and their lives."

Athenaca: "There's still so much to learn, and each discovery brings us closer to understanding the full tapestry of human history. It's a never-ending journey of exploration and discovery."

Jones: "I'm looking forward to learning more about these topics. They give a new perspective on who we are and where we come from."

Athenaca: "And that curiosity, Jones, is the essence of science. Keep asking questions and seeking answers. It's the path to deeper knowledge and understanding."

Out of Africa Theory:

The "Out of Africa" theory posits that all modern humans originated from a common African ancestor. As populations migrated out of Africa, they encountered diverse environments, leading to varying selective pressures on skin color.

Adaptation to New Environments: Human migration patterns show how populations adapted to different climates. In colder, low-UV regions, lighter skin evolved to facilitate vitamin D synthesis. In contrast, populations in high-UV areas retained darker skin to protect against sun damage.

Genetic Evidence - Genetic Markers and Ancestry: Genetic markers such as haplogroups provide insights into human migration and the evolution of skin color. Ancient DNA studies reveal how genetic variations in skin color genes correlate with historical migration patterns.

Comparative Studies: Comparative studies of modern and ancient populations highlight the adaptive significance of skin color. For instance, the genetic diversity within African populations shows various skin colors adapted to different UV levels.

Case Study: The Neanderthal Influence- Background: Neanderthals, an extinct hominin species, interbred with early modern humans.(Pavid, 2016). This interbreeding introduced genetic variants that influenced skin color in contemporary non-African populations.

Genetic Contributions: Genomic studies reveal that Neanderthal DNA contributed to variations in skin color, hair color, and other traits in modern humans. These genetic contributions highlight the complex interplay between different hominin species in shaping human diversity.

Health Implications: Neanderthal-derived genetic variants have been linked to skin and hair traits, influencing susceptibility to UV damage and vitamin D synthesis. Understanding these genetic influences provides insights into human adaptation and health.

Color Distribution:

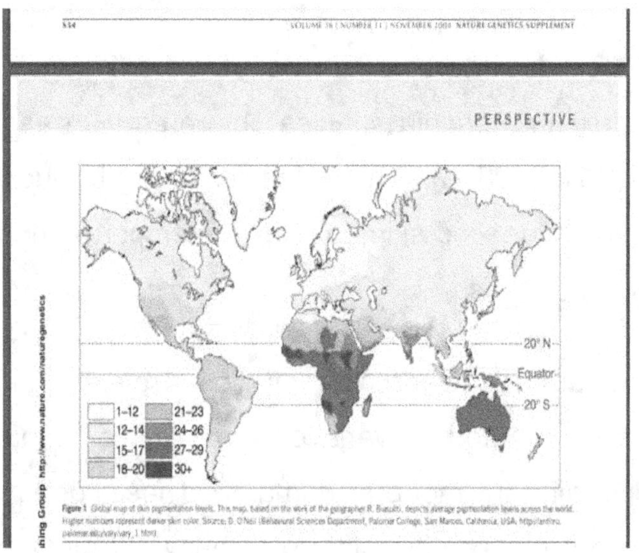

This is a map showing the Global skin color distribution of native populations. The colors on the map are based on the 36-tone chromatic scale devised by Austrian anthropologist Felix von Luschan to assess the unexposed skin of human populations. The higher numbers represent darker skin color. The original data was compiled by Biasutti in 1941. doi: 10.1371/journal.pone.0022103.g002; Taken from: (Dimasi et al., 2011)

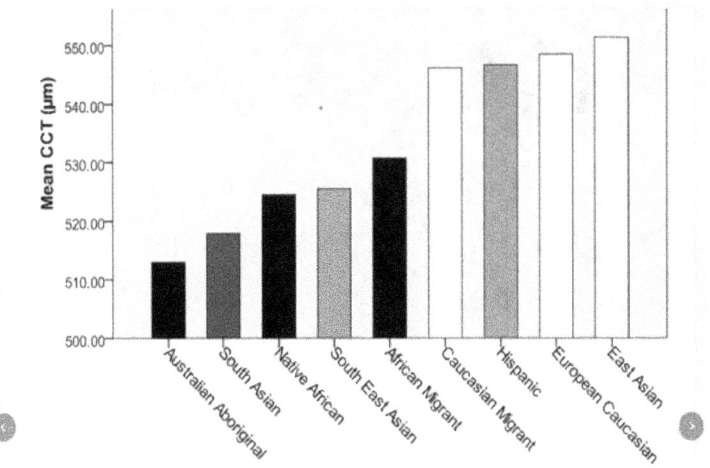

Taken from(Dimasi et al., 2011) Graphical representation of the human CCT meta-analysis results. (A) Mean CCT of each ethnic group. Colours indicate the tone of skin pigmentation according to the chart devised by Biasutti, 1941 (see Figure 1) (B) Mean CCT of the Dark Skin (524.6633.6 mm, n = 16,472) and Light Skin (548.4634.1 mm, n = 14,152) groups based on the skin colour of the ethnic groups in Figure 1A. There was a significant difference between the groups (p,0.001). doi: 10.1371/journal.pone.0022103.g003

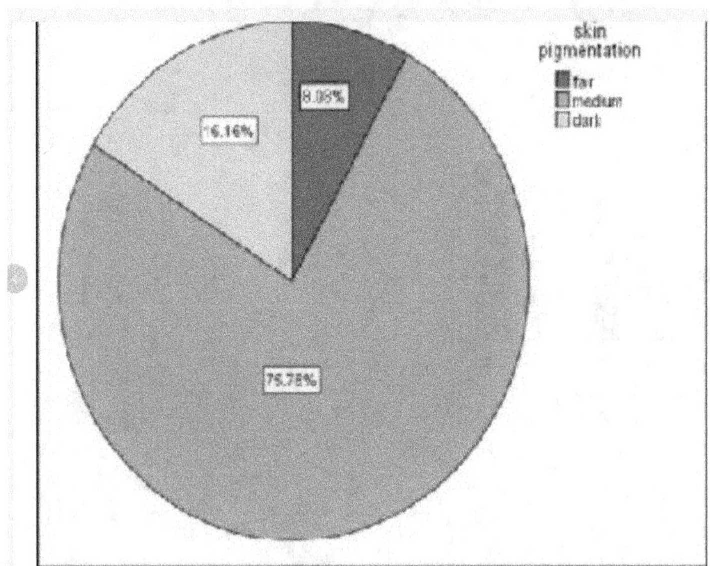

The above pie chart represents the percentage of skin color in patients, 76 percent, which Belongs to medium skin tone (Green). 16 percent are dark-skinned patients (Brown), and only 8 percent have fair skin tones (Blue) Taken from(Kaarthikeyan, 2021)

Regardless of these variations, all humans share a common ancestor who lived in Africa, so we all carry traces of our evolutionary history in our skin color.

The evolution of human skin color is a fascinating example of how our bodies have adapted to different environments over time. By understanding the genetic and environmental factors that have shaped our skin color, we can better appreciate the diversity of human populations worldwide(Jablonski and Chaplin, 2017).

Chapter 4: Future Directions in Skin Color Research

Advances in Genetics and Skin Color Studies - CRISPR-Cas9 and Gene Editing: CRISPR-Cas9 technology offers precise gene-editing capabilities, enabling researchers to study the genetic basis of skin color and its health implications. This technology holds potential for treating pigmentation disorders and understanding the genetic underpinnings of skin color.

Ethical Considerations

The use of gene-editing technologies raises ethical questions. Ensuring responsible use involves addressing potential risks, such as unintended genetic consequences and the implications for human diversity. Public engagement and moral frameworks are crucial for guiding these advancements.

Personalized Medicine

Tailoring Treatments to Genetic Profiles

Personalized medicine involves tailoring healthcare based on individual genetic profiles. Understanding the genetic basis of skin color can inform customized approaches to preventing and treating skin-related health issues.

Public Health Strategies

Addressing Health Disparities

Understanding the genetic and environmental factors influencing skin color can help address health disparities. Public health strategies should consider the diverse needs of different populations, promoting equitable access to healthcare and preventive measures.

Educational Initiatives

Educational initiatives can raise awareness about the importance of skin color in health. These initiatives should emphasize skin color's evolutionary and genetic basis, promoting an understanding that educational Initiatives can raise awareness about the importance of skin color in health. These initiatives should emphasize the evolutionary and genetic basis of skin color, promoting an understanding that'

Public Health Strategies

Educational initiatives can raise awareness about the importance of skin color in health. These initiatives should emphasize skin color's evolutionary and genetic basis, promoting an understanding that transcends social prejudices and highlights the scientific and medical significance. By fostering knowledge and appreciation for the diversity of human skin color, we can contribute to a more inclusive and equitable society.

Case Study - Public Health Campaigns

Background: Public health campaigns have successfully raised awareness about various health issues. These campaigns can be tailored to address skin color and health, emphasizing the need for sun protection, vitamin D supplementation, and regular skin checks.

Campaign Example: Sun Safety for All A campaign focused on sun safety could provide a tailored **Impact.** Such campaigns can significantly impact public awareness and behavior, reducing the incidence of skin cancer and vitamin D deficiency across diverse populations. Public health initiatives can address the unique needs of different groups and promote overall health and well-being by providing targeted information and resources.

Advice for different skin types could emphasize the importance of sunscreen use for individuals with lighter skin and the need for adequate sun exposure and vitamin D supplementation for those with darker skin.

Jones: "Athenaca, the advances in genetics have transformed our understanding of human skin color, haven't they?"

Athenaca: "Absolutely, Jones. Recent progress in genetics has shed light on the evolutionary origins of skin color and how it has evolved through natural selection. These discoveries highlight the complex interplay between genetics, environment, and adaptation."**(Liu, Bitsue and Yang, 2024).**

Jones: "So, multiple genes determine our skin color, each contributing to melanin production. This explains the wide variety of skin tones we see globally."

Athenaca: "Correct. By studying these genes, scientists have traced the origins of human skin color back to our earliest ancestors in Africa. The first humans evolved with dark skin to protect against the intense UV radiation in tropical regions."**(Jablonski and Chaplin, 2017).**

Jones: "As humans migrated from Africa to different parts of the world, their skin color changed in response to new environmental pressures, right? This process is called convergent evolution."

Athenaca: "Exactly. In areas with less sunlight, such as northern Europe, natural selection favored lighter skin tones to allow for better absorption of UV radiation and production of vitamin D. This adaptive process led to a wide range of skin colors in human populations worldwide."**(Jablonski, Chaplin, 2017).**

Jones: "I read that other factors, like diet and lifestyle, influence skin color. For example, foods rich in carotenoids can enhance skin pigmentation and protect against UV damage."

Athenaca: "Yes, that's true. The interplay between genetics and environmental factors is crucial in understanding the evolution of human skin color. For instance, the MC1R gene significantly determines melanin type, with specific variants leading to red hair and fair skin. This is crucial for lighter skin pigmentation in European populations."**(MedlinePlus, 2024).**

Jones: "These genetic discoveries challenge long-held beliefs about race and identity. By uncovering the mechanisms behind skin pigmentation, scientists are advancing our understanding of human diversity."

Athenaca: "Indeed, Jones. Our skin color is a testament to the remarkable resilience and adaptability of the human species. As we unravel the mysteries of our evolutionary past, we gain deeper insights into the complexity of human diversity."**(Jablonski and Chaplin, 2017).**

Jones: "Speaking of the future, gene editing technology like CRISPR-Cas9 can potentially alter human skin color. This could reduce the risk of skin cancer and other UV-related damage."

Athenaca: "Gene editing indeed holds immense potential. CRISPR-Cas9 allows for precise modifications to the DNA sequence, enabling scientists to add, remove, or alter genetic material. This technology could revolutionize preventive healthcare by enhancing melanin production, thus offering protection against UV radiation and reducing the incidence of skin cancer and photoaging(*SIRT7 gene knockout using CRISPR/Cas9 system enhances melanin production in the melanoma cells - PubMed*, no date).

Jones: "But there are significant ethical and social implications, right? Modifying fundamental traits like skin color could lead to many ethical dilemmas."

Athenaca: "Yes, the ethical implications of gene editing for skin color modification are profound. While the potential health benefits are considerable, we must cautiously navigate these possibilities. Understanding the evolutionary context of skin color is essential to preserve human diversity and avoid unintended consequences."**(Jablonski and Chaplin, 2017).**

Jones: "So, even as scientists explore genes involved in melanin production, like TYR, OCA2, and SLC24A5, there's a need for extensive research and clinical trials to ensure safety and efficacy before applying these findings to humans."

Athenaca: "Absolutely. We need to consider the long-term impacts on human diversity and adaptability. Our skin color diversity is a testament to our species' ability to thrive in various environments. Preserving this diversity is crucial for cultural and social reasons and the resilience it provides against changing environmental conditions."**(MedlinePlus, 2024)**.

Jones: "Integrating gene-editing technology into clinical practice will require a balanced approach. Public engagement and education will be crucial to building trust and understanding about the capabilities and limitations of gene editing."

Athenaca: "Yes, fostering open dialogue and establishing robust ethical standards will help ensure that advancements in gene editing contribute positively to society. By considering the scientific, ethical, and social dimensions, we can harness the benefits of gene editing while safeguarding equity and diversity."**(MedlinePlus, 2024)**.

Jones: "Ultimately, our goal should be to deepen our understanding of skin color and its implications for health and society. This knowledge can help create more effective health interventions and challenge discriminatory practices."

Athenaca: "Precisely, Jones. By tracing the evolution of human skin color from Africa to everywhere, we uncover the intricate story of our species and the profound ways we have adapted to diverse environments. Gene editing holds the potential to reshape our understanding of human health and disease, but we must navigate these possibilities with careful consideration."**(MedlinePlus, 2024).**

Jones: "Through a comprehensive and inclusive approach, we can realize the benefits of gene editing while respecting the rich diversity of human skin color and promoting a more equitable society."

Athenaca: "Well said, Jones. By continuing research and education, we empower ourselves to create a future where diversity is seen as a strength and scientific advancements contribute to the well-being of all individuals."

Jones: "Athenaca, can you explain the TYR and OCA2 genes and their functions in simpler terms?"

Athenaca: "Sure, Jones. Let's break it down. TYR and OCA2 are both genes that play important roles in determining our skin, hair, and eye color."**(MedlinePlus, 2024)**

Jones: "Okay, let's start with TYR. What does it do?"

Athenaca: "The TYR gene makes an enzyme called tyrosinase. This enzyme is crucial for producing melanin, the pigment that gives color to our skin, hair, and eyes. Think of tyrosinase as a key ingredient in the recipe for melanin."(*TYR gene: MedlinePlus Genetics*, no date)

Jones: "So, without tyrosinase, we wouldn't have melanin?"

Athenaca: "Exactly. A problem with the TYR gene can lead to a lack of melanin production, resulting in conditions like albinism, where people have very light skin, hair, and eyes.**"**

Jones: "Got it. Now, what about the OCA2 gene?"

Athenaca: "The OCA2 gene helps regulate the amount and type of melanin produced in our bodies. It's like a control panel that fine-tunes melanin production. Specifically, it influences how much melanin is present in our skin, hair, and eye cells"(*Is eye color determined by genetics?: MedlinePlus Genetics*, no date)

Jones: "So, does it work together with TYR?"

Athenaca: "Yes, it does. While TYR is crucial for making melanin, OCA2 helps determine how much melanin gets made and stored in the cells. Variations in the OCA2 gene can affect skin, hair, and eye color, contributing to the diversity of these traits among people."**(MedlinePlus, 2024).**

Jones: "So, in simple terms, TYR is like the factory that makes melanin, and OCA2 is like the manager that decides how much melanin the factory should produce?"

Athenaca: "That's a great way to put it, Jones. Together, these genes help create the wide range of colors we see in human skin, hair, and eyes.**"(MedlinePlus, 2024).**

Jones: "Thanks, Athenaca. That helps me understand how these genes shape our appearance."

Jones: "Athenaca, can you explain CRISPR-Cas9 to me simply?"

Athenaca: "Of course, Jones. Let's think of CRISPR-Cas9 as a pair of molecular scissors and a GPS combined. It's a tool that scientists use to edit genes in our DNA precisely.**"(MedlinePlus, 2024).**

Jones: "Molecular scissors and a GPS? How does that work?"

Athenaca: "Imagine our DNA is a long string of instructions written in a particular code. Sometimes, there are mistakes or parts we want to change. CRISPR-Cas9 helps us find those specific parts and make precise changes.**"(MedlinePlus, 2024).**

Jones: "So, how does it know where to cut?"

Athenaca: "That's where the GPS part comes in. CRISPR stands for 'Clustered Regularly Interspaced Short Palindromic Repeats,' which is a fancy way of saying it includes a special guide RNA. This guide RNA is like a GPS that leads the Cas9 protein, the molecular scissors, to the exact spot in the DNA where we want to cut."**(MedlinePlus, 2024).**

Jones: "And what does Cas9 do once it gets there?"

Athenaca: "Cas9 is the scissors part. Once the guide RNA brings Cas9 to the right spot, Cas9 cuts the DNA at that specific location. After the cut is made, the cell's natural repair processes kick in. Scientists can use this repair process to add, remove, or replace pieces of DNA at the site of the cut."**(MedlinePlus, 2024).**

Jones: "So, CRISPR-Cas9 can fix mistakes in our DNA or even add new instructions?"

Athenaca: "Exactly. It's a powerful tool for editing genes, which means it can potentially correct genetic defects, treat diseases, and even modify physical traits like skin color. However, because it's so powerful, many ethical considerations and safety tests must be addressed before using it widely in humans."**(MedlinePlus, 2024).**

Jones: "Wow, that sounds like it could change much about medicine and how we treat diseases."

Athenaca: "It has the potential to revolutionize many areas of science and medicine. But like with any powerful tool, we must use it carefully and responsibly."

Jones: "Thanks, Athenaca. That makes CRISPR-Cas9 a lot easier to understand!"

Conclusion

Jones: "Athenaca, the conclusion of our discussion emphasizes the importance of caution and responsibility in gene editing, especially when it comes to modifying skin color."

Athenaca: "Indeed, Jones. While gene editing holds immense potential for reducing health risks like skin cancer and enhancing our understanding of human biology, it also raises significant ethical and social concerns that we must address."

Jones: "So, the scientific community needs to be careful and consider the evolutionary context of skin color. Why is that so important?"

Athenaca: "It's crucial because our skin color has evolved over thousands of years in response to different environmental conditions. By understanding this evolutionary background, we can better appreciate the complexity of our genetic makeup and avoid oversimplifying the implications of genetic modifications."

Jones: "That makes sense. We also need to establish robust ethical standards. What kind of standards are we talking about?"

Athenaca: "We need guidelines that ensure gene editing is used responsibly and equitably. This includes considering the potential long-term impacts on human diversity and ensuring that the technology isn't used to reinforce social inequalities or discriminatory practices."

Jones: "So, fostering open dialogue is key to this process?"

Athenaca: "Absolutely. By engaging a broad range of stakeholders—scientists, ethicists, policymakers, and the public—we can ensure that diverse perspectives are considered. This helps build trust and ensures the technology is developed and applied to benefit all individuals."

Jones: "Through continued research and education, we can deepen our understanding of skin color and its health implications. How does this help society?"

Athenaca: "It empowers us to create more effective health interventions and challenge discriminatory practices. By highlighting skin color's biological and evolutionary aspects, we can foster a world where diversity is seen as a strength, not a source of division."

Jones: "Tracing the evolution of human skin color from Africa to everywhere uncovers the intricate story of our species. How does this knowledge impact our view on human adaptability and resilience?"

Athenaca: "It shows us how humans have thrived in diverse environments by adapting to different conditions. This resilience and adaptability are at the core of our shared humanity. Recognizing this helps us appreciate the rich tapestry of human diversity."

Jones: "Gene editing technology has the potential to reshape our understanding of health and disease. What should we keep in mind as we navigate these possibilities?"

Athenaca: "We must carefully consider the scientific, ethical, and social dimensions involved. Only through a comprehensive and inclusive approach can we fully realize the benefits of gene editing while safeguarding the principles of equity and diversity that are fundamental to our shared humanity."

Jones: "So, in conclusion, it's all about balancing the benefits with the risks and ensuring that advancements in gene editing contribute positively to society."

Athenaca: "Exactly, Jones. By fostering open dialogue, establishing robust ethical standards, and continuing research and education, we can harness the potential of gene editing technology to promote well-being and respect the rich diversity of human skin color. This balanced approach will help us create a more equitable and inclusive future."

Chapter 5: Relationship between Health and Skin Colour - Its Role in Vitamin D Synthesis.

Jones stood in the park, feeling the sun warm his face. He knew that this warmth wasn't just pleasant—it was essential. The sunlight on his skin was helping his body produce vitamin D, a vital nutrient for his bones and immune system. He wondered how people with different skin colors might experience this process differently and how it affected their health.

Vitamin D and Health

Vitamin D deficiency can lead to several health issues. Vitamin D synthesis begins in the skin under UVB radiation, converting 7-dehydrocholesterol to vitamin D3. This then transforms in the liver to 25-hydroxyvitamin D [25(OH)D] and finally in the kidneys to the active form 1,25-dihydroxyvitamin D [1,25(OH)2D]. A Martineau et al. (2017) meta-analysis found that vitamin D supplementation can significantly reduce the risk of acute respiratory infections, underscoring its crucial role in immune function.

Based on what we've read in the above chapters, skin color plays a crucial role in health due to its impact on the body's ability to produce vitamin D. When exposed to sunlight, the skin synthesizes vitamin D, which is essential for calcium absorption, bone growth, and immune function(Jablonski, Chaplin, 2017).

Melanin, the pigment responsible for our skin color, significantly influences the efficiency of vitamin D production. Melanin absorbs UVB radiation, providing a natural sunscreen effect. While this protective mechanism reduces the risk of sunburn and skin cancer, it also diminishes the amount of UVB radiation available for vitamin D synthesis.

What is Vitamin D?

Vitamin D is a fat-soluble vitamin that promotes calcium absorption, regulates bone growth, and plays a role in immune function. The skin synthesizes vitamin D when exposed to sunlight. However, dietary intake becomes essential if you spend much time indoors or live in a high-latitude region. Fatty fish, fish oils, egg yolks, butter, and liver are excellent dietary sources of vitamin D. However, obtaining sufficient vitamin D from diet alone can be challenging since natural sources are limited. Consequently, vitamin D deficiency is relatively standard. Fortunately, many food manufacturers fortify products like milk, margarine, and breakfast cereals with vitamin D. Additionally, supplements are widely used(WebMD, 2024).

Jones: Hi, Athenaca. I read this interesting article about vitamin D and its role in autoimmune diseases, but I'm having trouble understanding some of it. Could you help me understand it better?

Athenaca: Of course, Jones. I'd be happy to help. What specifically are you struggling with?

Jones: The article mentions diseases like MS, SLE, and RA. Can you explain these in more straightforward terms?

Athenaca: Certainly. MS, or multiple sclerosis, is a condition where the immune system mistakenly attacks the protective covering of nerve fibres, disrupting communication between your brain and the rest of your body. SLE stands for systemic lupus erythematosus, a disease where the immune system attacks its tissues, causing widespread inflammation and tissue damage. RA, or rheumatoid arthritis, is an autoimmune disorder where the immune system attacks the joints, leading to painful swelling and potential joint deformity**(Dupuis et al., 2021):**

Jones: That makes more sense. The article also talks about vitamin D's role in the immune system. How does it work exactly?

Athenaca: Vitamin D is crucial for a well-functioning immune system. The active form, 1,25-dihydroxyvitamin D, influences innate and adaptive immune systems. It helps reduce inflammation and encourages the immune system to tolerate itself rather than attacking the body's cells.

Jones: And how does it do that?

Athenaca: Vitamin D binds to the vitamin D receptor, or VDR, found in various immune cells. This binding affects the expression of specific genes and modulates how the immune cells respond to threats.

Jones: The article also mentions a link between vitamin D deficiency and autoimmune diseases. How are they connected?

Athenaca: When the body lacks sufficient vitamin D, its ability to regulate the immune system is compromised. This deficiency has been associated with an increased risk of developing autoimmune diseases like MS, RA, and SLE. Interestingly, these diseases are more common in women.

Jones: Why are these diseases more common in women?

Athenaca: One key factor is estrogen, a hormone higher in women. Estrogen can interact with vitamin D, enhancing its immune-regulating effects. This interaction can lead to different immune responses in men and women.

Jones: So, estrogen makes vitamin D more effective in women?

Athenaca: Yes, estrogen boosts the expression of VDR and reduces the enzymes that deactivate vitamin D. This means that vitamin D's immune-modulating effects are more pronounced in women.

Jones: And how does vitamin D affect those autoimmune diseases specifically?

Athenaca: Let's break it down by each disease. For MS, women have a higher risk of developing it but generally fare better than men once they have it. Vitamin D deficiency increases the risk of

MS, especially in women. Supplementation can benefit women, particularly those with higher estrogen levels.

Jones: What about RA and SLE?

Athenaca: Vitamin D can help reduce inflammation and disease severity in RA by modulating the immune response. Vitamin D deficiency is linked to more active disease. Estrogen's role in RA is complex; it can promote and reduce inflammation, depending on the context.

For SLE, estrogen tends to exacerbate the disease, which is why pregnancy can make SLE symptoms worse due to hormone changes. Vitamin D deficiency is common in SLE patients and is associated with higher disease activity, although the effectiveness of supplementation varies across studies.

Jones: So, should people with these conditions take vitamin D supplements?

Athenaca: Vitamin D could be a valuable addition to treating autoimmune diseases, especially for women, due to its interaction with estrogen. However, more research is needed to determine the best supplementation strategies based on sex and age.

Jones: Got it. Thanks, Athenaca. This helps a lot!

Athenaca: You're welcome, Jones. I am always happy to help you understand these complex topics.

This review highlights the importance of considering sex and gender differences in vitamin D-related immune modulation, potentially paving the way for personalized therapeutic approaches in autoimmune diseases.

 It was Monday, and Jones had just come from school and had dinner when he saw Athenaca passing by his home from work. He quickly ran after him.

Jones: Hi, Athenaca. I've been reading a lot lately. This morning, I read this article about common skin conditions for people of color, and I was hoping you could explain it to me in simpler terms.

Athenaca: Absolutely, Jones. Let's go through the main points together. What would you like to start with?

Jones: The article mentions skin cancer first. Is it different for people with darker skin?

Athenaca: Yes, it is. Skin cancer, particularly melanoma, is less common in people of color but tends to be more dangerous. It's often diagnosed late because it usually appears in areas not typically exposed to the sun, like under nails, on the soles of the feet, or around the genitals. This late diagnosis can make it more dangerous. Regular self-checks and sunscreen with at least SPF

30 can help with early detection and prevention:**(Common Skin Conditions for People of Color, no date)**.

Jones: I see. And what about acne?

Athenaca: Acne affects everyone, regardless of skin color. However, for people with darker skin, acne can leave behind dark spots called hyperpigmentation. It's important to treat acne early and avoid picking at it to prevent these spots from worsening **(Common Skin Conditions for People of Color, no date)**.

Jones: Eczema was also mentioned. How does it appear on darker skin?

Athenaca: Eczema can look a bit different on darker skin. Instead of the usual red, itchy patches on lighter skin, eczema on darker skin might appear as dry, flaky areas over deep pink, purple, or brown/grey patches. To manage eczema, it's best to use gentle skin care products, avoid hot showers, and avoid fragranced products **(Common Skin Conditions for People of Color, no date)**.

Jones: What are keloids?

Athenaca: Keloids are overgrowths of scar tissue that can become quite large. They are more common in African Americans and can be itchy or tender. Steroid injections can help reduce their size and discomfort. Considering any procedures that affect the skin, like piercings, it's essential to weigh the pros and cons because these can trigger keloid formation **(Common Skin Conditions for People of Color, no date)**.

Jones: The article also talks about melasma. What is that?

Athenaca: Melasma causes brown patches on the face. It's often influenced by hormonal changes, such as those during pregnancy or from birth control pills. Sunscreens that contain zinc or titanium are recommended to protect the skin, and treatments can include topical creams and cosmetic procedures to lighten the patches **(Common Skin Conditions for People of Color, no date)**.

Jones: And vitiligo?

Athenaca: Vitiligo causes white patches on the skin due to a loss of pigment. This is more noticeable in people with darker skin and can significantly impact their quality of life. Treatment options include topical steroids, ointments, and phototherapy. Sunscreen protects these areas from sunburn **(Common Skin Conditions for People of Color, no date)**.

Jones: It sounds like seeing a dermatologist is essential for these conditions.

Athenaca: Definitely. The article emphasizes the importance of consulting with a dermatologist for skin changes. Dermatologists can provide comprehensive care and treatment for these conditions, ensuring better management and improved quality of life **(Common Skin Conditions for People of Color, no date)**.

Jones: Thanks, Athenaca. This helps clarify things!

Athenaca: You're welcome, Jones. I'm glad I could help! Always feel free to ask if you have more questions.

Vitamin D Metabolism—Detailed Mechanisms: Vitamin D metabolism involves complex processes. UVB radiation converts 7-dehydrocholesterol in the skin to vitamin D3, which is then hydroxylated in the liver to 25-hydroxyvitamin D (Calcidiol). This is further hydroxylated in the kidneys to form 1,25-dihydroxyvitamin D (calcitriol), the active form. This hormone regulates calcium and phosphate homeostasis in the body, which is crucial for maintaining bone health and overall metabolic functions.

Factors Influencing Vitamin D Levels Several factors influence vitamin D levels, including geographic location, season, skin color, age, and body mass index (BMI). For instance, individuals living at higher latitudes with less sunlight exposure, older adults, and those with higher BMI are at increased risk of vitamin D deficiency. Understanding these factors helps tailor public health recommendations for diverse populations.

Expanded Narrative: Addressing Vitamin D Deficiency - Strategies for Different Populations: Effective strategies for addressing vitamin D deficiency must consider the needs of different populations. For instance, darker-skinned individuals living in northern latitudes might require higher vitamin D supplements than those with lighter skin. Public health guidelines should reflect these differences to ensure optimal health outcomes for all.

Case Study - Vitamin D Supplementation in Pregnancy

Background: Vitamin D deficiency during pregnancy can have severe consequences for the mother and the developing foetus. Adequate vitamin D levels are crucial to support maternal health and foetal development.

Health Implications Pregnant women with vitamin D deficiency are at higher risk of preeclampsia, gestational diabetes, and preterm birth. Adequate vitamin D levels support foetal bone development and reduce the risk of neonatal complications.

Intervention Strategies Healthcare providers often recommend vitamin D supplements for pregnant women, particularly those at higher risk of deficiency. The recommended daily allowance (RDA) for pregnant women is around 600 IU, but some may require higher doses based on individual assessments. Regular testing of vitamin D levels during pregnancy can help ensure that women maintain optimal levels.

Case Study - Vitamin D Deficiency in Different Ethnic Groups

Background: Research indicates that vitamin D deficiency prevalence varies significantly across different ethnic groups due to differences in skin pigmentation and cultural practices related to sun exposure. For instance, studies have shown higher rates of deficiency among African American and South Asian populations compared to Caucasians.

Health Outcomes Ethnic disparities in vitamin D levels have been linked to various adverse health outcomes. For example, African American populations have higher incidences of hypertension and certain cancers, which some studies suggest may be partially related to lower vitamin D levels.

Intervention Strategies

Targeted public health interventions are necessary to address these disparities. This could include community-based education programs about the importance of vitamin D, subsidized access to vitamin D-rich foods and supplements, and policies encouraging safe sun exposure practices.

Diagnosis:

Jones: Hi, Athenaca. I realized we didn't talk much about diagnosing vitamin D deficiency last time. Can you explain how that's done?

Athenaca: Sure, Jones. Diagnosing vitamin D deficiency involves measuring serum 25-hydroxyvitamin D levels in the blood. This is the most reliable marker of vitamin D status in the body.

Jones: Who needs to be tested for vitamin D deficiency?

Athenaca: High-risk individuals should be tested. This includes people with limited sun exposure, those with darker skin, older adults, individuals with certain medical conditions, and those who are obese. It's also essential for people living in northern latitudes with limited sunlight, especially during winter.

Jones: What's considered an optimal level of vitamin D?

Athenaca: The optimal serum level of 25-hydroxyvitamin D is debated among experts. However, the International Society for Clinical Densitometry and the International Osteoporosis Foundation recommend a level of 50 nmol/1 for bone health at all ages(*Vitamin D | International Osteoporosis Foundation*, no date)

Jones: Are there differences in how different races metabolize vitamin D?

Athenaca: There are significant differences in mineral metabolism among different races. For instance, African Americans tend to have higher bone density and a lower risk of fractures compared to other races. This means they might have different vitamin D requirements. Unfortunately, the effects of calcium and vitamin D supplementation in non-White populations haven't been thoroughly studied or reported, so more research is needed in this area.

Jones: What about the risks of having too much vitamin D?

Athenaca: There isn't enough data to precisely define the maximum safe upper level of serum 25-hydroxyvitamin D. However, levels above 100 ng/mL can pose a risk of toxicity, primarily due to secondary hypercalcemia, which is an excess of calcium in the blood(**Sizar et al., 2024**).

Jones: How is secondary hypercalcemia related to vitamin D?

Athenaca: Secondary hypercalcemia can occur when there's too much vitamin D in the body, leading to increased calcium absorption from the gut. For patients diagnosed with vitamin D deficiency, it's crucial to monitor for secondary hyperparathyroidism by measuring parathyroid hormone and serum calcium levels. This helps ensure that treatment with vitamin D doesn't lead to excessive calcium levels.

Jones: So, regular testing is essential?

Athenaca: Absolutely. Regular testing helps ensure that vitamin D levels are within a safe and effective range, especially for those at higher risk of deficiency. It allows for timely adjustments in sunlight exposure, diet, or supplementation.

Jones: Thanks for explaining this, Athenaca. I now understand how vitamin D deficiency is diagnosed.

Athenaca: You're welcome, Jones. It's always good to have a thorough understanding of these topics. If you have more questions, feel free to ask!

Prevention:

Jones: Hi, Athenaca. I also read this article about the best sources and supplements for vitamin D, and I could use some help understanding the details.

Athenaca: Sure, Jones. Let's go through the main points together. Where would you like to start?

Jones: The article mentions sunlight as a primary source of vitamin D. How does that work?

Athenaca: Sunlight is the primary source of vitamin D. When your skin is exposed to UVB rays from the sun, it produces vitamin D. For many people, just 5 to 15 minutes of sun exposure, 2 to 3 times a week, can be enough. However, this varies depending on skin type, location, season, and time of day. People with lighter skin need less sun exposure than those with darker skin**(WebMD, 2024).**

Jones: So, we need to balance sun exposure with the risk of skin cancer, right?

Athenaca: Exactly. Getting enough sunlight for vitamin D and protecting your skin from too much UV exposure is essential, as too much UV exposure can increase the risk of skin cancer.

Jones: What about dietary sources? What foods are good for vitamin D?

Athenaca: A few good dietary sources of vitamin D. Fatty fish and seafood like salmon, mackerel, sardines, and tuna are among the best. For instance, a serving of cooked salmon provides about 570 IU of vitamin D, more than half the daily value many health authorities recommend.

Jones: That sounds good. Are there any other sources?

Athenaca: Yes, cod liver oil is another excellent source. Just one teaspoon offers around 450 IU of vitamin D. Additionally, many countries fortify foods like milk, breakfast cereals, and orange juice with vitamin D. Dairy and plant-based milk alternatives, such as almond, soy, and oat milk, are often fortified with about 100-150 IU per cup**(WebMD, 2024).**

Jones: What if someone can't get enough vitamin D from sunlight or diet? Are supplements a good option?

Athenaca: Supplements are a practical option for those who may not get enough vitamin D from sunlight and diet. There are two main types: vitamin D3 (cholecalciferol) and vitamin D2 (ergocalciferol).

Jones: What's the difference between D3 and D2?

Athenaca: Vitamin D3 is generally considered more effective at raising blood levels of vitamin D. It's typically derived from lanolin (sheep's wool) or fish oil. On the other hand, vitamin D2 is a plant-based option suitable for vegans. It's derived from irradiated yeast and mushrooms. While D2 is less potent and not as well absorbed as D3, it's still a viable option**(WebMD, 2024).**

Jones: How should someone choose a supplement?

Athenaca: When choosing a supplement, look for ones certified by third-party organizations like USP (United States Pharmacopeia), NSF International, or ConsumerLab. These certifications ensure that the supplement contains what the label claims and is free from harmful contaminants. Also, consider the appropriate dosage—most adults need about 600-800 IU daily, but some may require higher doses, so it's best to consult a healthcare provider**(WebMD, 2024).**

Jones: Are there any brands you recommend?

Athenaca: Some reputable brands that meet rigorous testing standards include Nature Made, Nordic Naturals, and Carlson. Always opt for well-known and trusted brands.

Jones: The article also talks about monitoring vitamin D levels. How important is that?

Athenaca: It's essential, especially for those at higher risk of deficiency. A simple blood test can reveal if you need to adjust your sun exposure, diet, or supplementation. High-risk individuals should have their serum 25-hydroxyvitamin D levels measured to assess their vitamin D status.

Jones: What's the optimal level of vitamin D?

Athenaca: The optimal serum level of 25-hydroxyvitamin D is a topic of debate, but the International Society for Clinical Densitometry and the International Osteoporosis Foundation suggest that older individuals maintain a minimum level of 30 ng/mL to reduce the risk of falls and fractures. Levels above 100 ng/mL might be toxic, causing secondary hypercalcemia. It's also essential to check for secondary hyperparathyroidism by measuring parathyroid hormone and serum calcium levels**(Sizar et al., 2024).**

Jones: What's the best way to maintain adequate vitamin D levels?

Athenaca: Combining all three sources—sunlight, diet, and supplements—can ensure optimal vitamin D levels tailored to individual needs and circumstances. Always consult healthcare providers when deciding on supplementation, especially for higher doses or if there are any pre-existing health conditions.

Jones: Thanks, Athenaca. This clarifies things for me!

Choosing Supplements:

Jones: Hi, Athenaca. I read this article about the best sources and supplements for vitamin D, and I could use some help understanding the details.

Athenaca: Sure, Jones. Let's go through the main points together. Where would you like to start?

Jones: The article mentions sunlight as a primary source of vitamin D. How does that work?

Athenaca: Sunlight is the primary source of vitamin D. When your skin is exposed to UVB rays from the sun, it produces vitamin D. For many people, just 5 to 15 minutes of sun exposure, 2 to 3 times a week, can be enough. However, this varies depending on skin type, location, season, and time of day. People with lighter skin need less sun exposure than those with darker skin**(WebMD, 2024).**

Jones: So, we need to balance sun exposure with the risk of skin cancer, right?

Athenaca: Exactly. Getting enough sunlight for vitamin D and protecting your skin from too much UV exposure is essential, as too much UV exposure can increase the risk of skin cancer.

Jones: What about dietary sources? What foods are good for vitamin D?

Athenaca: A few good dietary sources of vitamin D. Fatty fish and seafood like salmon, mackerel, sardines, and tuna are among the best. For instance, a serving of cooked salmon provides about 570 IU of vitamin D, more than half the daily value many health authorities recommend.

Jones: That sounds good. Are there any other sources?

Athenaca: Yes, cod liver oil is another excellent source. Just one teaspoon offers around 450 IU of vitamin D. Additionally, many countries fortify foods like milk, breakfast cereals, and orange juice with vitamin D. Dairy and plant-based milk alternatives, such as almond, soy, and oat milk, are often fortified with about 100-150 IU per cup**(WebMD, 2024).**

Jones: What if someone can't get enough vitamin D from sunlight or diet? Are supplements a good option?

Athenaca: Supplements are a practical option for those who may not get enough vitamin D from sunlight and diet. There are two main types: vitamin D3 (cholecalciferol) and vitamin D2 (ergocalciferol).

Jones: What's the difference between D3 and D2?

Athenaca: Vitamin D3 is generally considered more effective at raising blood levels of vitamin D. It's typically derived from lanolin (sheep's wool) or fish oil. On the other hand, vitamin D2 is a plant-based option, suitable for vegans, and derived from irradiated yeast and mushrooms. While D2 is less potent and not as well absorbed as D3, it's still a viable option**(Vitamin D2 vs. D3: What's the Difference? 2018).**

Jones: How should someone choose a supplement?

Athenaca: When choosing a supplement, look for ones certified by third-party organizations like USP (United States Pharmacopeia), NSF International, or ConsumerLab. These certifications ensure that the supplement contains what the label claims and is free from harmful contaminants. Also, consider the appropriate dosage—most adults need about 600-800 IU daily, but some may require higher doses, so it's best to consult a healthcare provider.

Jones: Are there any brands you recommend?

Athenaca: Some reputable brands that meet rigorous testing standards include Nature Made, Nordic Naturals, and Carlson. Always opt for well-known and trusted brands.

Jones: The article also talks about monitoring vitamin D levels. How important is that?

Athenaca: It's essential, especially for those at higher risk of deficiency. A simple blood test can reveal if you need to adjust your sun exposure, diet, or supplementation. High-risk individuals should have their serum 25-hydroxyvitamin D levels measured to assess their vitamin D status**(Sizar et al., 2024)**.

Jones: What's the optimal level of vitamin D?

Athenaca: The optimal serum level of 25-hydroxyvitamin D is a topic of debate, but the International Society for Clinical Densitometry and the International Osteoporosis Foundation suggest that older individuals maintain a minimum level of 30 ng/mL to reduce the risk of falls and fractures. Levels above 100 ng/mL might be toxic, causing secondary hypercalcemia. It's also essential to check for secondary hyperparathyroidism by measuring parathyroid hormone and serum calcium levels**(Sizar et al., 2024).**

Jones: I read that African Americans tend to have higher bone density and a lower risk of fractures. How does that relate to vitamin D?

Athenaca: Yes, African Americans generally have higher bone density and a lower risk of fractures compared to other races. However, the effects of calcium and vitamin D supplementation in non-White populations haven't been thoroughly studied. It's essential to tailor vitamin D recommendations to individual needs and consider these differences in mineral metabolism.

Jones: What's the best way to maintain adequate vitamin D levels?

Athenaca: Combining all three sources—sunlight, diet, and supplements—can ensure optimal vitamin D levels tailored to individual needs and circumstances. Always consult healthcare providers when deciding on supplementation, especially for higher doses or if there are any pre-existing health conditions.

Jones: Thanks, Athenaca. This clarifies things for me!

Athenaca: You're welcome, Jones. I'm glad I could help! If you have more questions, feel free to ask.**Vitamin D Deficiency - causes, symptoms, and impacts:**

Jones: Hi, Athenaca. I read about vitamin D deficiency and wanted to discuss it in more detail, especially its causes, symptoms, and impacts.

Athenaca: Of course, Jones. Let's dive into it. What do you want to start with?

Jones: What exactly is vitamin D deficiency?

Athenaca: Vitamin D deficiency occurs when your body doesn't have enough vitamin D. This vitamin is crucial for various bodily functions, including bone health, immune system support, and muscle function.

Jones: dark-skinned people are more susceptible to vitamin D deficiency. Why is that?

Athenaca: That's right. People with dark skin have more melanin, which reduces the skin's ability to produce vitamin D from sunlight. The National Institutes of Health (NIH) notes that individuals with darker skin are likelier to have lower vitamin D levels than those with lighter skin. Common symptoms of vitamin D deficiency include fatigue, muscle weakness, bone pain, and an increased risk of infections. These symptoms can be subtle and easily overlooked, so people with dark skin need to monitor their vitamin D levels.

Jones: Does ethnicity play a role in vitamin D deficiency?

Athenaca: Yes, it does. Research shows that African Americans, Hispanics, and South Asians are more likely to have lower vitamin D levels compared to Caucasians. This is partly due to differences in skin pigmentation and how their bodies metabolize vitamin D.

Jones: How about fair-skinned individuals? Do they have the same risk?

Athenaca: Fair-skinned individuals have less melanin, so they can absorb UVB radiation more efficiently and produce vitamin D more effectively. However, this increased efficiency also raises the risk of sunburn and skin cancer if proper sun protection isn't used. While they are generally less likely to develop vitamin D deficiency, they can still be at risk if they live in areas with limited sunlight or have lifestyles that limit sun exposure.

Jones: How should people balance sun exposure and skin protection?

Athenaca: It's essential to strike the right balance. The American Academy of Dermatology recommends limiting direct sun exposure during peak hours (10 a.m. to 2 p.m.), wearing protective clothing, and applying broad-spectrum sunscreen with an SPF of 30 or higher. Individuals with darker skin may need more sun exposure to achieve optimal vitamin D levels. In contrast, fair-skinned individuals should get 10 to 15 minutes of direct sun exposure two to three times a week before applying sunscreen**(Watson, King, and PhD, no date)**.

Jones: I read something about vitamin D and COVID-19. Can you explain that?

Athenaca: Certainly. Several studies suggest that vitamin D deficiency may increase the risk and severity of COVID-19. For instance, LL Benskin's review in "Frontiers in Public Health" discusses preliminary evidence indicating that vitamin D deficiency might elevate COVID-19 risks. Other studies, like those by R Kumar et al. and M Kohlmeier, highlight vitamin D's role in modulating the immune response and potentially reducing the severity of COVID-19. Overall, maintaining adequate vitamin D levels could be a public health strategy to reduce the impact of COVID-19.

Jones: What are the symptoms and causes of vitamin D deficiency?

Athenaca: Symptoms in adults can be subtle and include muscle cramps, mood changes, fatigue, and more. Severe deficiency in children can lead to rickets, causing abnormal growth patterns, muscle weakness, and joint deformities. In adults, it can cause fatigue, bone pain, muscle weakness, and mood changes like depression. Causes include inadequate vitamin D intake, insufficient sunlight exposure, and the body's inability to properly absorb or utilize vitamin D. Certain medical conditions, weight-loss surgeries, and medications can also lead to deficiency.

Jones: Which medical conditions and medications contribute to vitamin D deficiency?

Athenaca: Conditions like cystic fibrosis, Crohn's, and celiac disease can hinder vitamin D absorption. Obesity and kidney and liver diseases also affect how vitamin D is processed and converted into its active form. Weight-loss surgeries like gastric bypass can impair nutrient absorption, necessitating lifelong supplementation. Medications like laxatives, steroids, cholesterol-lowering, seizure-preventing, specific tuberculosis, and weight-loss drugs can lower vitamin D levels.

Jones: What are the health risks of vitamin D deficiency?

Athenaca: The health risks are significant. For bone health, vitamin D is essential for calcium absorption, maintaining bone density, and preventing osteoporosis. In the immune system, it helps modulate responses and reduce the risk of autoimmune diseases. Muscle function can be impaired, leading to weakness and an increased risk of falls. There's evidence linking vitamin D to mood regulation and cardiovascular health. Deficiency can lead to rickets in children, Osteomalacia in adults, impaired immune function, increased cancer risk, and complications during pregnancy.

Jones: This information is comprehensive. Thanks for explaining everything, Athenaca.

Athenaca: You're welcome, Jones. It's important to understand these health issues thoroughly. If you have any more questions, feel free to ask!

Chapter 6

CULTURAL IDENTITIES AND SOCIAL DYNAMICS

How Skin Color Has Shaped Cultural Identities and Social Dynamics Throughout History

Jones: Athenaca, I've been thinking about how much our identities are shaped by things we can't control, like our skin color. It seems like such a superficial trait, but it significantly impacts our lives and societies. How has skin color influenced cultural identities and social dynamics throughout history?

Athenaca: That's a profound question, Jones. The story of skin color is indeed intertwined with our history, cultures, and social structures. To understand this fully, we must return to ancient civilizations and work our way to the present.

Jones: Let's start with ancient civilizations, then. How did they view skin color?

Athenaca: In ancient Egypt, for instance, skin color was depicted in art, showing a diverse society where different shades were standard and seemed to be a part of their social fabric. The Egyptians didn't use skin color to segregate people as strictly as later societies did. Their society focused more on social roles and hierarchies based on occupation and wealth.

Jones: So, they didn't see skin color like we do now?

Athenaca: Not precisely. While they acknowledged differences, these weren't the primary markers of identity. Moving on to the Greeks and Romans, their attitudes were complex. They often associated lighter skin with the elite who stayed indoors and darker skin with laborers who worked outside. Yet, social mobility existed, and one's status could change regardless of skin tone.

Jones: That's interesting. What about during the Middle Ages and the Renaissance?

Athenaca: During the Middle Ages, European views on skin color were shaped by religious and philosophical beliefs. Darker skin was sometimes seen as exotic or even linked to negative traits due to a lack of understanding and the influence of religious interpretations. By the Renaissance, with the age of exploration, Europeans began categorizing people based on skin color more systematically. This laid the groundwork for the racial hierarchies that justified colonialism and slavery.

Jones: Ah, colonialism and slavery. These must have had a significant impact on perceptions of skin color.

Athenaca: Absolutely. Colonialism and the transatlantic slave trade entrenched the idea that lighter skin was superior. European colonizers used skin color as a primary marker to classify and control people, with darker-skinned individuals often viewed as inferior and enslaved. This period significantly shaped global attitudes toward skin color, embedding deep-seated prejudices that persist to this day.

Jones: That explains a lot about the historical context. But how did these perceptions evolve into cultural identities?

Athenaca: Skin color became central to cultural identity in many societies. For example, in India, the caste system often correlated lighter skin with higher status, a notion that persists even now. Similarly, in East Asia, fair skin has long been associated with beauty and status. Art, literature, and media perpetuated these cultural norms, reinforcing the association between skin color and social value.

Jones: It's like these cultural norms became self-perpetuating. But were there any cultures that saw darker skin positively?

Athenaca: Yes, indeed. Many African cultures traditionally celebrate darker skin as a mark of beauty and strength. The Maasai people, for example, admire dark skin for its health and vitality. These cultural perspectives offer a different narrative in which darker skin is revered rather than marginalized.

Jones: It seems that skin color has also influenced social dynamics. How did this happen in more recent history, like the United States?

Athenaca: The United States provides a stark example of how skin color has shaped social dynamics. The history of slavery and segregation left deep scars. The "one-drop rule" enforced a rigid racial boundary, where any African ancestry made one Black, reinforcing discrimination against darker-skinned individuals. Even after civil rights progress, colorism persisted, with lighter-skinned individuals often receiving preferential treatment in various spheres of life, from employment to media representation.

Jones: That must have also created many internal divisions within communities.

Athenaca: Precisely. Colorism created hierarchies within marginalized communities, often leading to internal conflicts. This issue is not unique to the United States; many countries with colonial histories struggle with colorism today. It affects people's opportunities and self-esteem, perpetuating inequality.

Jones: What about health implications? Does skin color affect how societies address health issues?

Athenaca: Skin color has significant health implications, especially regarding UV protection and vitamin D synthesis. Darker skin provides better protection against UV radiation but can lead to vitamin D deficiency in low sunlight regions.

Conversely, lighter skin is more prone to UV damage but synthesizes vitamin D more efficiently. These differences necessitate tailored public health strategies to address the specific needs of different populations.

Jones: That sounds like a complex balance to manage. How do cultural practices fit into this?

Athenaca: Cultural practices affect how skin health is perceived and managed. For instance, the Danish concept of hygiene, emphasizing coziness and well-being, promotes self-care practices that are beneficial for skin health. Similarly, feng shui, which focuses on harmony and balance, can reduce stress and promote a healthy environment, indirectly supporting skin health.

Jones: It's fascinating how interconnected everything is. But what about the future? Are there any advancements on the horizon that could change how we view and manage skin color-related issues?

Athenaca: Advances in genetic research, particularly technologies like CRISPR, hold promise for treating pigmentation disorders. These could potentially correct genetic mutations responsible for conditions like albinism and vitiligo. Moreover, there is a growing awareness of the need to address health disparities related to skin color, which could lead to more equitable healthcare policies and practices.

Jones: We seem to have come a long way, but there's still much to do.

Athenaca: Indeed, Jones. Understanding skin color's historical and cultural context is crucial for addressing today's challenges. By recognizing the impact of these dynamics, we can work towards a more inclusive and equitable society.

Jones: Thank you, Athenaca. This has been enlightening. I now have a much deeper understanding of how skin color has shaped and continues to shape our world.

Athenaca: You're welcome, Jones. Remember, the journey of understanding is ongoing, and by learning about the past, we can better navigate the future.

Jones: Let's investigate how these dynamics occur in specific historical contexts. For instance, how did the Spanish colonizers perceive and treat indigenous people in the Americas based on their skin color?

Athenaca: Like many Europeans, the Spanish colonizers operated under a framework that equated lighter skin with superiority. They viewed the darker-skinned indigenous populations as inferior and in need of conversion to Christianity and European ways of life. This belief justified their colonization efforts, leading to the subjugation and exploitation of millions of indigenous people. The Spanish caste system, or "castes," was a complex hierarchy that ranked individuals based on their racial heritage, heavily influencing social and economic opportunities.

Jones: It sounds like the caste system institutionalized racism. Did it have lasting effects?

Athenaca: Yes, the effects of the caste system are still felt today in many Latin American countries. The legacy of these racial hierarchies continues to influence social dynamics, where lighter skin is often associated with higher status and better opportunities. This ongoing impact can be seen in the disparities in wealth, education, and political power that persist in these regions.

Jones: It's disheartening to see how deeply entrenched these issues are. What about in Africa, where European colonizers imposed their rule in the 19th century?

Athenaca: European colonization in Africa devastated the continent's social structures. Colonizers imposed racial hierarchies that privileged lighter-skinned Europeans and marginalized darker-skinned Africans. These hierarchies were enforced through governance, education, and economic exploitation. The division and marginalization exacerbated ethnic tensions and disrupted traditional social systems.

Jones: How did Africans respond to these imposed racial structures?

Athenaca: Africans resisted colonization in various ways, from armed resistance to cultural and intellectual movements. Leaders like Nelson Mandela and Kwame Nkrumah played pivotal roles in the fight against colonial rule and racial oppression. Post-independence, many African nations have worked to reclaim their cultural identities and address the legacy of colonialism, though challenges remain.

Jones: How do these historical influences manifest in the modern context?

Athenaca: In contemporary society, the historical influences of skin color continue to shape social dynamics. For instance, the Black Lives Matter movement highlights ongoing racial disparities and seeks to address the systemic racism that disproportionately affects people of darker skin tones. Similarly, movements like #MeToo have shed light on how intersecting identities, including race and gender, affect individuals' experiences of discrimination and violence.

Jones: Skin color is more than just a physical trait; it's deeply woven into the fabric of our societies. How do we move forward in addressing these complex issues?

Athenaca: Moving forward requires a multifaceted approach. Education is critical to understanding the historical and cultural context of skin color and helps dismantle prejudiced beliefs. Policy changes are crucial, ensuring that laws and practices promote equity and inclusion. Fostering open dialogues about race and skin color can help bridge divides and promote mutual understanding.

Jones: What role do individuals play in this process?

Athenaca: Individuals have a significant role to play. People can contribute to change by challenging their biases and supporting inclusive policies.

The following Saturday afternoon, Jones sat on a weathered wooden bench in the lush garden at the back of his home, leafing through the article assigned by his mentor. His eyes traced the lines of "Pathways to Skin Color Stratification: The Role of Inherited (Dis)Advantage and Skin Color Discrimination in Labor Markets" by Maria Abascal and Denia Garcia. A gentle breeze rustled the pages as though urging him to reflect deeper. Soon, he saw Athenaca approaching, her presence always a beacon of wisdom.

Jones: (looking up with a thoughtful expression) Athenaca, this article by Abascal and Garcia is quite revealing. It delves into how skin color impacts labor market outcomes. But there's so much to unpack here. Can we discuss it?

Athenaca: (smiling warmly as she sits beside him) Of course, Jones. Let's explore its depths together. Where would you like to begin?

Jones: The authors talk about "inherited (dis)advantage." It's intriguing how they link skin color with socio-economic status across generations. Can we start there?

Athenaca: (nodding) Certainly. Inherited (dis)advantage refers to the advantages or disadvantages passed down from generation to generation. Skin color plays a crucial role in this because of historical and systemic inequalities. Darker-skinned individuals often face more barriers, limiting their socio-economic mobility compared to their lighter-skinned counterparts. This creates a cycle of disadvantage.

Jones: (thoughtfully) Right. The article mentions how these disparities are not just personal but institutional. Discrimination in education, housing, and healthcare cumulatively affects labor market outcomes. It's like the odds are stacked against darker-skinned individuals from birth.

Athenaca: Exactly. Abascal and Garcia emphasize these systemic barriers. The institutional discrimination perpetuates a cycle where darker-skinned individuals start at a disadvantage and have fewer opportunities to advance, reinforcing the socio-economic gap across generations.

Jones: (pausing) And then there's the aspect of skin color discrimination within the labor market itself. The authors provide examples of how employers often favor lighter-skinned candidates, assuming they possess better qualities. It's unsettling.

Athenaca: Yes, it's a harsh reality. This bias, often unconscious, stems from deep-rooted societal prejudices. Employers might perceive lighter skin as more competent or trustworthy, affecting hiring decisions, salary, and career advancement opportunities. Though subtle, these prejudices profoundly impact individuals' careers and lives.

Jones: (leaning back) It's almost as if skin color becomes a silent, unwelcome determinant of one's professional destiny. The authors argue that lighter-skinned individuals are more likely to be hired and promoted even with equal qualifications. How do we counteract such ingrained biases?

The next day, Jones and Athenaca sat in the quiet library, surrounded by the scent of old books and the soft hum of the air conditioning. Jones looked up from his notes, his face a mix of curiosity and confusion. Athenaca noticed and leaned in, ready to discuss.

Athenaca: You seem deep in thought, Jones. What's on your mind?

Jones: I've been reading about different stories of racism and redemption, and I'm trying to piece it all together. I read about Byron Widner, Wendy Kelly, and even a case of a Black professor accused of discriminating against white students. Each story is so different, yet they all deal with the theme of racism. Can we discuss each one in detail?

Athenaca: Absolutely. Each story offers a unique perspective on racism. Let's start with Byron Widner's story.

Byron Widner's Transformation

Byron Widner was deeply involved in the white supremacist movement as a member of the Vinlanders Social Club, a violent skinhead group. For 16 years, Widner was immersed in a world of hate, engaging in numerous violent acts and spreading a message of white supremacy. His body was a canvas of hate, covered in tattoos symbolizing his racist beliefs.(*Reformed skinhead endures agony to remove tattoos*, no date)

Widner's journey to redemption began when he met Julie, a woman who had also been involved in the white power movement but had left it behind. They married, and with her support, Widner started to see the flaws in his beliefs. He wanted a better life for his family, free from hate and violence. However, escaping his past was not easy. His tattoos made it impossible to hide his former life, and he faced threats from his former associates.

The pivotal moment came when Widner connected with Daryle Lamont Jenkins, an activist who helps individuals leave extremist groups. Jenkins guided Widner through deradicalization and provided the support he needed. With financial assistance from the Southern Poverty Law Centre, Widner underwent 24 painful procedures to remove his tattoos. Each session was a step away from his past and a commitment to his new life(*Reformed skinhead endures agony to remove tattoos*, no date).

Widner's story is a powerful testament to the possibility of change. It shows that even those deeply entrenched in hate can find redemption with the proper support and a genuine desire to transform. His journey highlights the importance of empathy, understanding, and the willingness to help those seeking to leave a life of violence and prejudice behind.

Jones: That's incredible. It's amazing how someone can turn their life around so drastically. But then there's Wendy Kelly. Her experiences are quite different but equally compelling.

Wendy Kelly's Struggle Against Racism: Wendy Kelly's story is a poignant illustration of the subtle and overt forms of racism that Black individuals face daily. From childhood to adulthood, Wendy encountered numerous instances of racial prejudice that shaped her understanding of the world.

As a child, Wendy was often asked why her skin looked ashy, a term used to describe the appearance of dry skin on Black people. This seemingly innocent question was loaded with ignorance and insensitivity, making Wendy self-conscious about her appearance. Such experiences were the beginning of her long journey through a world that often saw her as different and less than because of her skin color(*"Is This Because I'm Black?": A Story of Racial Discrimination | TLNT*, no date)

In her professional life, Wendy faced systemic racism in the workplace. Despite her qualifications and hard work, she was consistently underpaid compared to her white colleagues. One particularly jarring incident occurred during a job interview for a receptionist position. The hiring manager expressed relief at being able to pronounce her name, assuming she was white based on her name alone. This blatant display of racial bias left Wendy feeling devalued and frustrated(*"Is This Because I'm Black?": A Story of Racial Discrimination | TLNT*, no date).

Her experiences in corporate America were no different. Wendy discovered that a less experienced white colleague earned significantly more than her. When she confronted her manager about the pay disparity, he admitted that he had tried to get her a raise but was unsuccessful. This incident reinforced the systemic nature of racial discrimination in the workplace and the ongoing struggle for equality.

Wendy's story highlights the everyday racism that many Black people face. It shows how systemic issues and individual prejudices intersect, creating a challenging environment for those simply trying to live and work on equal terms. Her resilience and determination to confront these challenges are inspiring and underscore the need for continued efforts to address racial inequalities.

Jones and Athenaca were sitting under a large oak tree in the schoolyard. Jones looked thoughtful, his notebook on his lap. Athenaca noticed and decided to start the conversation.

Athenaca: What's on your mind today?

Jones: I've been reading an article by Rodolfo Mendoza-Denton about racism against whites(Mendoza-Denton, 2011). It's complex. Can we discuss it?

Athenaca: Absolutely. Mendoza-Denton's work is fascinating. What stood out to you?

Jones: The article discusses how whites are beginning to engage in collective actions, like courses and rallies, against perceived racism. It seems like what minority groups have done historically. He also talks about stereotypes and how they affect interactions between racial groups.

Athenaca: That's an important point. Mendoza-Denton notes that stereotypes about whites—seeing them as discriminatory or intolerant—can lead to efforts to appear overly likable. On the other hand, minorities often must combat stereotypes of being seen as incompetent, leading them to focus on gaining respect. These divergent goals can cause misunderstandings during interactions(Mendoza-Denton, 2011).

Jones: Yes, he mentions that these crossed signals can result in negative feelings because both parties feel misunderstood. They're trying so hard to counteract stereotypes that they misinterpret each other's intentions.

Athenaca: Exactly. This is particularly problematic in interracial interactions. If one person is trying to be liked and the other is trying to be respected, their efforts can seem insincere or unfriendly to the other. This dynamic can perpetuate the cycle of inequality and prevent genuine understanding and connection (Mendoza-Denton, 2011).

Jones: Mendoza-Denton also points out that even stereotypes against historically dominant groups can contribute to inequality. It's not just about who has power but how these stereotypes hinder our ability to relate and collaborate effectively.

Athenaca: Indeed. Small steps, like open communication and genuine efforts to understand one another(Mendoza-Denton, 2011). Stereotypes create barriers that prevent us from seeing each other as individuals. They can keep us from working together, hiring each other, or even forming friendships. Breaking these barriers requires

Jones: So, it's about creating spaces where people can connect without the weight of these stereotypes. That sounds challenging but necessary.

Athenaca: It is challenging but essential for addressing structural inequalities. By recognizing and addressing these stereotypes, we can level the playing field and foster more meaningful and equitable relationships.

Jones: Thank you, Athenaca. These discussions have helped me see things more clearly.

Athenaca: You're welcome, Jones. Combating these biases requires multifaceted approaches. First, raising awareness about these unconscious biases through workplace education and training programs is essential. Second, implementing and enforcing anti-discrimination laws and policies can provide a framework for fairness. Lastly, fostering inclusive environments where diversity is genuinely valued can gradually shift these prejudiced mindsets.

Jones: (nodding) Education and policy enforcement sound like starting points, but changing mindsets seems like the most formidable challenge. How do we ensure that diversity is genuinely valued beyond just ticking boxes?

Athenaca: True, genuine inclusion goes beyond tokenism. It involves creating a culture where diverse voices are heard and valued. This can be achieved through mentorship programs, diverse leadership, and continuous dialogue about the benefits of diversity. People need to see diversity as an asset, not an obligation.

Jones: (smiling) I suppose you're right. Awareness is the first step. This discussion has given me a lot to think about. Thank you, Athenaca.

Athenaca: (patting his shoulder) Remember, knowledge is the key to unlocking change. Keep questioning, keep learning, and you'll find ways to make a difference.

Jones watched as Athenaca walked away, her words resonating in his mind. He looked back at the article, now seeing it as a study and a call to action. The journey towards equality was long, but he felt more equipped to contribute to the change with each conversation.

One bright sunny weekend, Jones was sitting on the porch, engrossed in more readings on the topic. He felt a tap on his shoulder and turned to see Athenaca holding a stack of books.

Jones: Athenaca, I want to discuss Dr Nina Jablonski's interview in Appalachian Today, "Insights on the impact of race and prejudice from Dr Nina Jablonski's interview."

Athenaca: Definitely, Jones. Dr Jablonski's program brings together a diverse group of scientists, social scientists, artists, and educators to address these entrenched racial issues. The goal is to rethink and reset societal views on race by creating new educational initiatives and modes of dialogue.

Jones: So, it's about changing how people think and talk about race?

Athenaca: Exactly. She believes that by bringing discussions about race into both polite and impolite company, we can start to dismantle the stereotypes that persist. It's challenging work because people often feel uncomfortable discussing race, but it's necessary for change.

Jones: That makes sense. She also talks about teaching race and genetics to young students. How does that help?

Athenaca: Dr Jablonski argues that understanding race's scientific and historical aspects from a young age can demystify it. By teaching children about the evolution of skin color and human history, we can prevent the formation of prejudiced views. Kids are naturally curious and open-minded, so early education on these topics can build a foundation for a more inclusive mindset.

Jones: It's like giving them the tools to understand and accept diversity before prejudices take root.

Athenaca: Precisely. When children learn about the natural and historical reasons for different skin colors, it becomes just another fact of life rather than a basis for division. This knowledge empowers them to question and resist prejudices they might encounter later.

Jones: She mentions a "minor revolution" in education. What does she mean by that?

Athenaca: She's calling for a fundamental change in how education addresses race. This means integrating these concepts into the curriculum from an early age, not as a separate subject, but as a natural part of learning about the world and human biology. It's about normalizing the discussion of race factually and openly.

Jones: That sounds like a significant shift from how things are taught. How realistic is this change?

Athenaca: It's ambitious but not impossible. It requires educators to be well-prepared and supported in teaching these topics. Dr Jablonski's efforts include developing curriculums and training teachers to handle these discussions effectively. It's a gradual process, but commitment can significantly change societal attitudes.

Jones: So, it's about creating an informed and open-minded generation?

Athenaca: Exactly. By thoroughly educating young people about the origins and implications of race, we hope to foster a society that values diversity and understands the harm of prejudice. Dr Jablonski's work is about laying the groundwork for this transformation.

Jones: (thoughtfully) I read an article that mentioned the concept of "intersectionality." How does this relate to skin color discrimination?

Athenaca: Intersectionality, a term coined by Kimberlé Crenshaw, refers to how different aspects of a person's identity—such as race, gender, class, and skin color(*Intersectional Self - FYS 101 - Research Guides at Syracuse University Libraries*, no date) — intersect and create unique experiences of discrimination and privilege. For example, a dark-skinned woman might face both racial and gender discrimination, which can compound and create unique challenges that a light-skinned man might not experience.

Jones: (leaning forward) That makes sense. So, addressing skin color discrimination isn't just about tackling one issue; it's about understanding how it intersects with other forms of discrimination.

Athenaca: Exactly. A holistic approach requires us to consider all these intersecting factors. It's about recognizing the complexity of individuals' experiences and creating solutions that address this complexity. For instance, in the labor market, policies must include various identities and experiences to be truly effective.

Jones: (pausing) Regarding policies, what effective strategies have been implemented to combat skin color discrimination in the labor market?

Athenaca: Several initiatives have addressed this issue. For example, some companies have implemented blind recruitment processes, where identifying information such as name and photo is removed from applications to reduce bias. Others have diversity training programs to raise awareness about unconscious biases. Additionally, some organizations have set diversity targets and quotas to ensure a more representative workforce.

Jones: (interested) Blind recruitment sounds promising. But how effective are these measures in the long run?

Athenaca: While these measures are steps in the right direction, their effectiveness varies. Blind recruitment can help reduce initial biases but doesn't address the more profound, systemic issues. Diversity training can raise awareness, but it needs to be ongoing and coupled with other initiatives to be truly impactful. Setting targets and quotas can help create a more diverse workforce, but ensuring that these individuals are supported and valued within the organization is crucial.

Jones: (thoughtfully) It's about creating a comprehensive approach that combines various strategies.

Athenaca: Exactly. Each solution must address the issue partially. It's about creating an environment where diversity is genuinely valued and systemic barriers are actively dismantled. This requires commitment and effort from all levels of an organization, from leadership to employees.

Jones: (sighing) It's challenging but not impossible. With the right mindset and dedication, we can create meaningful change.

Athenaca: Absolutely. Change is always possible but requires persistence and a willingness to confront uncomfortable truths. It's about moving beyond awareness to action and accountability.

Jones: I read Vibeke Sofie Sandager Rønnedal's article about racism in classic Nordic children's literature(*Racism in Classic*

Pieces of Nordic Children's Literature, no date). It's thought-provoking. Can we discuss it?

Athenaca: Of course, I'd be happy to. What aspects of the article stood out to you?

Jones: The article discusses how many beloved Nordic children's books contain racial prejudices that are either overt or subtly embedded. It's interesting to see how these books are republished with controversial content revised to fit contemporary views on race and racism. For example, Pippi Longstocking's father's title was changed from 'King of the Negroes' to 'King of the South Seas.'

Athenaca: That's a significant change. It reflects a broader effort to address historical racism in literature. What do you think about editing these books rather than preserving their original content?

Jones: That's what I find most intriguing. The article highlights a debate: Should we edit out racist elements to right historical wrongs, or does that risk sanitizing our history and neglecting essential aspects of our past?

Athenaca: It's a complex issue. Editing out racist elements can make these stories more appropriate for modern readers, promoting inclusivity and respect. On the other hand, it's important to remember and learn from our past, even the uncomfortable parts. Understanding historical context helps us recognize how far we've come and the work still needed.

Jones: The article also mentions that Nordic countries often view themselves as antiracist and post-racial societies. Yet, these debates reveal that there are still underlying issues related to their colonial past and racial understanding.

Athenaca: Exactly. This self-perception can sometimes mask the continuing relevance of racism and the need to address it. Revising children's literature, these societies are confronting their historical attitudes and working towards a more inclusive present. It's a delicate balance between correcting past wrongs and acknowledging them.

Jones: The discussion about the Icelandic nursery rhyme 'The Ten Little Negros' is another example. The illustrations were quite offensive, yet some defended the book as part of their cultural heritage. It shows how deeply ingrained these works are in people's identities.

Athenaca: Cultural heritage can be a powerful force. For many, these books are tied to childhood memories and national identity. Changing them can feel like erasing a part of that identity. However, it's also crucial to evolve and reflect contemporary values that reject racism and promote equality.

Jones: It's interesting how the article also touches on the backlash against political correctness and so-called 'reverse racism.' Some people see these revisions as unnecessary or an attack on free speech.

Athenaca: Yes, that's a common reaction. However, addressing racist content isn't about limiting free speech but about promoting respectful and inclusive discourse. It's about ensuring that our cultural artifacts do not sustain harmful stereotypes and are appropriate for all readers.

Jones: So, it's about balancing preserving cultural heritage and adapting to modern values of inclusivity and respect.

Athenaca: Precisely. It's a challenging but necessary task. By critically examining and revising these works, we can create a more inclusive cultural legacy while still acknowledging and learning from our past.

Jones: Thanks, Athenaca. This discussion helps me understand the nuances of this issue.

Athenaca: One critical difference is their focus on equality from a very early age. Their education systems emphasize inclusion and equal opportunity, ensuring that all children have access to high-quality education regardless of their background. Additionally, they have robust social safety nets that help reduce socio-economic disparities, which can mitigate the effects of inherited disadvantage.

Jones: (nodding) It sounds like a holistic approach is crucial. Addressing the issue from multiple angles is the most effective strategy.

Athenaca: Indeed. It's about creating an ecosystem where equality is ingrained in every aspect of society—from education and healthcare to housing and employment. Each sector plays a role in either perpetuating or dismantling these inequalities.

Jones: (Reflecting) Another article I read discusses the role of policy in combating skin color discrimination. What policies should governments implement to address this issue effectively?

Athenaca: Governments can implement various policies to address skin color discrimination. Anti-discrimination laws are fundamental, but they need to be enforced rigorously. Policies promoting equal education, healthcare, and housing access are also essential. Governments can also incentivize companies to adopt fair hiring practices and diversity programs. On a broader scale, social welfare policies that reduce economic inequality can help mitigate the impact of inherited disadvantage.

Jones: (enthusiastic) A lot can be done at the policy level. But how do we ensure these policies are effective and make a difference?

Athenaca: Monitoring and evaluation are essential. Policies need to be regularly reviewed to assess their impact and effectiveness. Governments and organizations should collect and analyze data to understand how these policies are working and where improvements are needed. Transparency and accountability are also crucial. Policymakers must be held accountable for the implementation and outcomes of these policies.

Jones: (thoughtfully) I see. It's about creating a continuous improvement cycle and ensuring policies evolve based on real-world outcomes.

Athenaca: Exactly. It's an ongoing process. Social attitudes and systemic structures don't change overnight, but persistent effort and commitment make progress possible.

Jones: (smiling) This gives me hope. There's so much to learn and do. I want to delve deeper into the psychological impacts of discrimination we discussed earlier. How can we support individuals who face these challenges?

Athenaca: Supporting individuals who face discrimination requires a multi-layered approach. On a personal level, providing access to mental health services is crucial. Counselling and therapy can help individuals cope with the stress and anxiety caused by discrimination. On an organizational level, creating safe and inclusive environments where individuals feel valued and supported is essential. Peer support groups and mentorship programs can also provide a sense of community and belonging.

Jones: (nodding) Mental health support seems critical, especially since the psychological impacts can be profound. How can organizations ensure they're providing adequate support?

Athenaca: Organizations must prioritize mental health as a diversity and inclusion strategy. This includes offering mental health resources, such as counselling services and employee assistance programs. It's also essential to foster a culture where mental health is openly discussed and employees feel comfortable seeking help. Training managers and leaders to recognize and address mental health issues can also make a significant difference.

Jones: (thoughtfully) It's about creating a culture of support and understanding, not just ticking off a box. Are there any specific examples of companies successfully integrating mental health support into their diversity initiatives?

Athenaca: Yes, some companies have been pioneers in this area. For example, Unilever has a comprehensive well-being program includes mental health support as a critical component. They offer mental health training for managers, provide access to counselling services, and promote a culture of openness around mental health. Similarly, Johnson & Johnson has initiatives focusing on mental health awareness and employee support.

Jones: (impressed) It's encouraging to see these examples. It shows that organizations can make a real difference in their employees' lives with the right approach. What about the role of education in addressing skin color discrimination? How can schools and universities contribute to this effort?

Athenaca: Education is a powerful tool for change. Schools and universities can play a crucial role by promoting diversity and inclusion early. This includes incorporating diverse perspectives into the curriculum, teaching students about the history and impact of discrimination, and fostering an inclusive environment where all students feel valued. Educators should be trained to recognize and address their biases and create a supportive learning environment for all students.

Jones: (thoughtfully) Education can seem to lay the foundation for a more inclusive society. By teaching children about diversity and inclusion early on, we can hopefully reduce biases and create a more equitable future.

Athenaca: Absolutely. Education can shape the attitudes and beliefs of future generations. It's about creating a culture of empathy, understanding, and respect for everyone, regardless of skin color.

Jones: (smiling) This conversation has been incredibly enlightening, Athenaca. I now have a much deeper understanding of the complexities of skin color discrimination and the various ways we can address it.

Athenaca: I'm glad to hear that, Jones. It's a complex issue, but we can make a difference with awareness, education, and action. Remember, every small step towards understanding and equality contributes to the more significant movement for change.

Jones: (determined) I'm committed to being part of that change. Thank you for guiding me through this critical topic, Athenaca.

Athenaca: (smiling warmly) Anytime, Jones. Keep questioning, learning, and striving for a more equitable world.

As Jones watched Athenaca walk away, her words resonated deeply within him. The journey towards understanding and combating skin color discrimination was far from over, but he felt more equipped and inspired to take meaningful action. He returned to his readings, determined to continue his quest for knowledge and change.

Later that evening, Jones sat at his desk, reflecting on the day's discussion. He drafted a plan for a school project to raise awareness about skin color discrimination and promote inclusion. As he outlined his ideas, he felt renewed purpose and determination.

Jones: (writing) Project Title: "Shades of Equality: Promoting Inclusion and Understanding of Skin Color Discrimination"

Objective: To raise awareness about the impact of skin color discrimination and promote a culture of inclusion and respect within the school community.

Activities:

1. **Educational Workshops:** Organize workshops that educate students and staff about the history and impact of skin color discrimination. Invite guest speakers from diverse backgrounds to share their experiences.
2. **Diversity Training:** Implement training programs for teachers and staff to recognize and address unconscious biases. Provide resources and tools to create an inclusive classroom environment.

3. **Peer Support Groups:** Establish peer support groups where students can share their experiences and provide mutual support. Create a safe space for open discussions about diversity and inclusion.

4. **Awareness Campaign:** Launch an awareness campaign that includes posters, social media, and school newsletters. Highlight stories of individuals who have overcome discrimination and promote positive representations of diversity.

5. **Inclusive Curriculum:** Work with teachers to integrate diverse perspectives into the curriculum. Ensure that history, literature, and social studies courses discuss skin color discrimination and its impact.

Evaluation:

- Conduct surveys to assess the effectiveness of the workshops and training programs.
- Gather feedback from students and staff about the peer support groups and awareness campaigns.
- Monitor changes in attitudes and behaviors towards diversity and inclusion within the school community.

Jones: (finishing his draft) This is just the beginning. We can create a more inclusive and understanding environment with dedication and effort.

Jones felt a sense of accomplishment as he saved his draft. He knew real change would require ongoing effort and collaboration, but he was ready to take the first step. Inspired by his discussion with Athenaca and the insights from Abascal and Garcia's article, he was determined to make a difference in his community.

Jones looked out the window as the night grew darker, feeling renewed hope and purpose. The path toward equality was long and challenging, but he was ready to walk it, one step at a time.

The next day, Jones shared his project plan with Athenaca, who was impressed by his initiative.

Athenaca: (reading the plan) This is an excellent initiative, Jones. I'm proud of your dedication and thoughtfulness. This project has the potential to make a significant impact.

Jones: (smiling) Thank you, Athenaca. Your guidance and our discussions have been incredibly inspiring. I'm excited to get started and make a difference.

Athenaca: (nodding) Remember, change begins with awareness and understanding. By fostering a culture of inclusion and respect, you're helping to create a more equitable future. Keep up the great work, and don't hesitate to reach out if you need any support.

Jones: (gratefully) Thank you, Athenaca. Your support means a lot to me. I'll keep you updated on the progress and any challenges we face.

Athenaca: (smiling warmly) I look forward to hearing about your journey. Remember, each step you take, no matter how small, contributes to the larger goal of equality and inclusion.

Jones left the meeting with a renewed sense of determination. He immediately began reaching out to fellow students and teachers, gathering a small team of like-minded individuals passionate about the project.

A few weeks later, the "Shades of Equality: Promoting Inclusion and Understanding of Skin Color Discrimination" project was underway. Jones and his team organized their first educational workshop, which students, teachers, and some parents attended. The guest speaker was Dr Elena Marquez, a respected sociologist specializing in race and ethnicity.

Dr Marquez: (addressing the audience) Good morning, everyone. It's an honor to be here and discuss the crucial topic of skin color discrimination. Our skin, the body's largest organ, should not determine our worth or opportunities. Yet, historically and even today, it often does. Let's delve into how we can change this.

The workshop was interactive, with students participating in discussions and activities designed to highlight unconscious biases and the impact of discrimination. One activity involved role-playing scenarios where students navigated prejudice and discrimination, fostering empathy and understanding.

Student 1: (participating in role-play) Seeing how these biases play out in everyday situations is eye-opening. I never realized how subtle yet pervasive they can be.

Student 2: (nodding) Me neither. This activity made me think about how I might unintentionally contribute to these biases and what I can do to change that.

Dr Marquez: (responding) That's precisely the point of these exercises. We can begin to address and dismantle these biases by recognizing and understanding them. Awareness is the first step towards change.

After the workshop, Jones and his team received positive feedback from attendees, who expressed a desire for more such events. Buoyed by the success, they moved forward with the other components of their project.

The next major initiative was the diversity training for teachers and staff. The training sessions were designed to help educators recognize and address their biases, creating a more inclusive classroom environment. They included discussions, case studies, and practical strategies for promoting diversity and inclusion.

Teacher 1: (reflecting during a session) I've never thought about how my teaching methods might unintentionally favor some students over others. This training is helping me see things from a different perspective.

Teacher 2: (agreeing) Same here. I'm learning new ways to ensure all my students feel valued and included, regardless of their background.

Facilitator: (leading the session) That's the goal. By being aware of our biases and actively working to counteract them, we can create a more equitable learning environment for all students.

Meanwhile, the peer support groups were gaining momentum. Students who had faced discrimination or felt marginalized found a safe space to share their experiences and support each other. The groups were facilitated by trained counsellors who provided guidance and resources.

Student 3: (speaking in a support group) It's comforting to know I'm not alone in my experiences. This group gives me a sense of belonging and strength to face challenges.

Counsellor: (nodding) You are not alone. Sharing your stories and supporting each other is a powerful way to heal and empower yourselves.

Jones was particularly proud of the awareness campaign. His team had created compelling posters and social media content highlighting the importance of diversity and shared stories of individuals overcoming discrimination. The campaign generated a lot of discussion within the school community and beyond.

Teacher 3: (commenting on a poster) These stories are incredibly inspiring. They remind us of the resilience and strength of individuals facing discrimination daily.

Parent: (reading a social media post) I'm glad my child's school addresses such an important issue. We need to have a conversation about it at home as well.

The final component of the project, integrating diverse perspectives into the curriculum, was more challenging but equally rewarding. Jones worked closely with teachers to identify opportunities to include discussions about skin color discrimination in history, literature, and social studies courses.

History Teacher: (planning a lesson) We can include more about the civil rights movement and the ongoing struggle for racial equality. Students need to understand that this is an ongoing issue, not just a historical one.

Literature Teacher: (agreeing) Absolutely. We can also introduce more diverse authors and stories that reflect different experiences and perspectives. This will help students see the world through different lenses.

Months passed, and the impact of the "Shades of Equality" project was becoming evident. The school environment was becoming more inclusive, and there was a noticeable shift in attitudes towards diversity and discrimination. Students and teachers were more aware of their biases and actively working to create a more equitable community.

One day, as Jones reviewed feedback from the latest workshop, Athenaca approached him with a proud smile.

Athenaca: (beaming) Jones, I've heard fantastic things about your project. The changes in the school are palpable. How are you feeling about everything?

Jones: (smiling) It's been a challenging but enriching journey. Seeing the positive impact and knowing we're making a difference is fulfilling. But I know there's still so much more to do.

Athenaca: (nodding) Indeed, the journey towards equality is ongoing. But you've laid a strong foundation. Your dedication and hard work have inspired many, including myself. What's next for you and the project?

Jones: (thoughtfully) We're planning to expand the project to other schools in the district. We've been documenting our process and outcomes to share our model with others. I also want to continue my studies in sociology and perhaps work on policy advocacy in the future.

Athenaca: (smiling warmly) That sounds like a beautiful plan. Your passion and commitment will undoubtedly lead to more positive changes. Remember, every step you take brings us closer to a more just and inclusive society.

Jones: (determined) Thank you, Athenaca. Your guidance has been invaluable. I'll keep pushing forward and striving for change.

As Jones walked through the school halls, he felt a deep sense of accomplishment and purpose. The "Shades of Equality" project had not only transformed his school but had also set him on a path toward lifelong advocacy and action. He knew that the journey was far from over, but he was making a difference with each step.

It's been three years since Jones started his project to educate people and combat discrimination in all its forms because of the color of a person's skin. Now, he's found himself standing in front of a large audience at an international conference on diversity and inclusion. He was now a respected sociologist and policy advocate known for combating skin color discrimination. As he began his speech, he reflected on the journey that had brought him here.

Jones: (addressing the audience) Good evening, everyone. It's an honor to be here today to discuss the crucial issue of skin color discrimination and the pathways to a more inclusive and equitable society. My journey began in high school with a project called "Shades of Equality." What started as a small initiative became a lifelong mission to create change.

The audience listened intently as Jones shared his experiences and insights. He spoke about the importance of education, policy, and cultural change in addressing discrimination. He highlighted the successes and challenges of his work, always emphasizing the need for persistence and collaboration.

Jones: (concluding his speech) Together, we can create a world where everyone, regardless of skin color, can thrive. This requires commitment, action, and a willingness to confront uncomfortable truths, but I believe in our collective power to make a difference. Thank you.

Jones felt a deep sense of fulfilment as the audience erupted into applause. Countless conversations, challenges, and triumphs had shaped his journey from a high school student to an international advocate. And it all began with a simple yet profound discussion with his mentor, Athenaca.

As he left the stage, Jones knew that the journey towards equality was far from over. But he was ready to continue the fight, inspired by the knowledge that every step contributed to the more significant movement for change, no matter how small.

Jones left the meeting with a renewed sense of determination.

Chapter 7: Conclusion

Throughout human history, skin color has been a powerful indicator of our species' remarkable ability to adapt to diverse environmental conditions. Far from being a mere superficial trait, skin color tells a complex story that intertwines evolution, health, genetic diversity, and cultural narratives. This intricate tapestry begins with our earliest ancestors in Africa and extends globally, highlighting skin pigmentation's biological underpinnings and societal implications.

Understanding skin color begins with recognizing its evolutionary significance. Human skin color evolved primarily due to varying sun ultraviolet (UV) radiation levels. Darker skin evolved as a protective mechanism in regions with intense UV radiation, such as near the equator. Melanin, the pigment responsible for skin color, absorbs and dissipates UV radiation, preventing DNA damage and reducing the risk of skin cancers. This adaptation was crucial for early humans' survival and reproductive success in these environments.

As humans migrated from Africa and settled in different parts of the world, their skin color adapted to the new environmental conditions. This process, known as convergent evolution, is evident in populations that developed similar traits independently due to similar environmental pressures. For instance, populations living in high UV environments, like those near the equator, evolved darker skin to protect against UV damage. Conversely, populations in low UV environments, such as northern Europe, developed lighter skin to optimize vitamin D synthesis, essential for bone health and immune function.

The genetic basis of skin color further illuminates this evolutionary narrative. Several essential genes, including MC1R and SLC24A5, play significant roles in melanin production and distribution. The MC1R gene influences whether melanocytes produce eumelanin (darker pigment) or pheomelanin (lighter pigment). Variants of the MC1R gene can lead to different shades of skin, hair, and eye color. For example, individuals with specific MC1R variants often have red hair and fair skin, a trait that evolved in response to the lower UV radiation levels in northern Europe.

The SLC24A5 gene, particularly influential in European populations, significantly impacts melanin synthesis and distribution. Variants of this gene are linked to lighter skin tones, a trait that evolved to adapt to environments with lower UV radiation. This genetic diversity underscores the crucial role of personalized medicine, which directs healthcare to individual genetic makeup. This approach acknowledges that people with different skin colors have varying susceptibilities to health issues like vitamin D deficiency and skin cancer, paving the way for more effective and equitable interventions.

Understanding the genetic factors behind skin color also helps address health disparities. For example, people with darker skin are more susceptible to vitamin D deficiency because melanin reduces the skin's ability to produce vitamin D from sunlight. On the other hand, individuals with lighter skin face a higher risk of UV-induced damage, which can lead to skin cancers. These insights underscore the critical need for tailored public health recommendations considering skin color and environmental factors to ensure more effective and equitable interventions.

Modern advancements in genetics, such as CRISPR-Cas9, offer a promising potential to address some of these health disparities. CRISPR-Cas9 is a powerful tool for gene editing that can correct genetic defects responsible for various diseases. However, its potential must be balanced with ethical considerations to prevent misuse. The responsible use of gene editing technologies necessitates the development of ethical guidelines and transparent public discourse. This open communication is crucial to ensure that scientific progress does not come at the cost of human diversity or equity.

The intersection of genetics, lifestyle, and environment is particularly relevant in addressing public health challenges. Urbanization and modern lifestyles have significantly altered our exposure to sunlight, impacting our ability to synthesize vitamin D. In many parts of the world, people spend most of their time indoors, leading to widespread vitamin D deficiency even in regions with abundant sunlight. This highlights the need for updated health strategies that include vitamin D supplementation and dietary adjustments to ensure adequate levels for all.

Our understanding of skin color also extends to its social and cultural dimensions. Throughout history, skin color has been a basis for social stratification and discrimination. Scientific knowledge can be crucial in dismantling these prejudices by highlighting the shared human story behind skin color variations. Education is critical in this regard. Promoting a science-based understanding of skin color can challenge and change long-held biases and stereotypes, paving the way for a more inclusive and equitable society.

Personal stories of individuals affected by racism and prejudice further illustrate the real-world impact of skin color. For instance, Byron Widner's transformation from a white supremacist to a reformed individual shows that even those deeply entrenched in hate can change with the proper support. Widner, a former member of the violent skinhead group Vinlanders Social Club, began his journey to redemption after meeting his wife, Julie, who had also left the white power movement. With the help of activist Daryle Lamont Jenkins and financial assistance from the Southern Poverty Law Centre, Widner underwent painful tattoo removal procedures to erase the symbols of his past. His story highlights the importance of empathy, understanding, and support in overcoming prejudice and hate.

Wendy Kelly's experiences with racism, from childhood to adulthood, illustrate the everyday challenges that Black individuals face. As a child, Wendy was often asked why her skin looked ashy, a term used to describe the appearance of dry skin on Black people. Such seemingly innocent questions were loaded with ignorance and insensitivity, making Wendy self-conscious about her appearance. In her professional life, Wendy faced systemic racism in the workplace, being consistently underpaid compared to her white colleagues. These experiences underscore the persistent nature of racism and the need for systemic reform to achieve equality.

The case of the Black professor accused of discriminating against white students adds another layer to the conversation. This story illustrates how accusations of racism can occur in any direction, highlighting the complexities of racial dynamics. It serves as a reminder that while systemic racism predominantly affects Black and minority communities, individual acts of prejudice can occur in any context.

We've learned about how different stereotypes but the same psychological processes can sustain conflict.

Understanding these nuances helps create a more comprehensive approach to combating racial discrimination and promoting equality.

Our research journey through the science of skin color has been enlightening in many ways. We've uncovered the intricate mechanisms behind skin color evolution and its implications for health and society. But there's still much to learn and many questions to answer. Future research should continue to explore the genetic basis of skin color and its interaction with environmental factors. Studying diverse populations will also provide a more comprehensive understanding of human adaptation and health.

As we look to the future, we must also consider the ethical dimensions of our work. Technologies like CRISPR-Cas9 hold great promise but also pose significant ethical challenges. We need robust frameworks to guide their use in a way that benefits humanity. Public engagement and interdisciplinary collaboration will be crucial in this endeavor. By involving diverse stakeholders, we can ensure that scientific advancements are aligned with societal values and contribute to the greater good.

In conclusion, our journey through the science of skin color has been a profound exploration of what it means to be human. It has shown us how our bodies have adapted to different environments, how genetics influence our health, and how societal factors shape our experiences. It has also highlighted the importance of viewing human diversity as a strength. We can promote a more inclusive and equitable world by understanding and embracing our differences.

GLOSSARY

- **Bone Density:** A measure of the strength of bones. Adequate vitamin D is crucial for maintaining healthy bone density.

- **Enzyme:** In biology, an enzyme is a type of protein that acts as a catalyst in biochemical reactions. Enzymes accelerate chemical reactions by lowering the activation energy needed for the reaction, allowing processes in the cell to happen more efficiently and faster.

- Eumelanin: A brown or black melanin that provides excellent protection against UV radiation.

- **Folate:** A type of B vitamin crucial for DNA synthesis and repair. Adequate melanin levels help protect folate from being broken down by UV radiation.

- Genetic Variants: Differences in the DNA sequence among individuals that can influence traits like skin color.

- Genome-wide association Studies (GWAS) are research studies that look for genetic variations across the entire genome that are associated with specific traits or diseases.

- **Hyperpigmentation:** A condition where patches of skin become darker than the surrounding skin, often due to excess melanin production.

- **Immune Function:** The body's ability to fight off infections and diseases. Vitamin D supports the immune system.

- **Keloids:** Raised scars that grow excessively at the site of a skin injury, more common in people with darker skin.

- **MC1R (Melanocortin 1 Receptor):** A gene that affects the type of melanin produced in the skin. Variants of this gene can result in different skin and hair colors.

- Melanin: A pigment produced by cells in the skin that gives color to the skin, hair, and eyes. It also protects against the harmful effects of the sun's ultraviolet (UV) radiation.

- **Melanocytes:** Specialized cells in the skin that produce melanin.

- **Natural Selection:** The process by which certain traits become more common in a population because they offer a survival or reproductive advantage.

- **Osteomalacia:** A condition in adults characterized by bone softening due to vitamin D deficiency. • Pheomelanin: A red or yellow melanin that offers less protection against UV radiation. •

Rickets: A bone disease in children caused by severe vitamin D deficiency, leading to soft and weak bones.

• SLC24A5 (Solute Carrier Family 24 Member 5) is a gene that influences skin color by affecting melanin production. It is associated with lighter skin in some populations.

• **Sunburn:** Skin damage caused by excessive exposure to UV radiation, which can lead to redness, pain, and sometimes peeling.

• **UV Radiation:** Ultraviolet light from the sun that can cause skin damage and increase the risk of skin cancer. It is necessary to produce vitamin D in the skin.

• **Vitamin D:** A nutrient essential for maintaining bone health and supporting the immune system. The skin produces it when exposed to sunlight.

• **Vitamin D Deficiency:** A condition with insufficient vitamin D in the body can lead to bone problems and weaken the immune system.

• **Vitiligo:** A condition where skin patches lose color due to the destruction of melanocytes.

Bibliography:

Bristol, U. of (no date) *Skin colour gives clues to health.* University of Bristol. Available at: https://www.bristol.ac.uk/news/2009/6658.html (Accessed: 24 June 2024).

Davies, G., Garami, A.R. and Byers, J. (2020) 'Evidence Supports a Causal Role for Vitamin D Status in Global COVID-19 Outcomes'. medRxiv, p. 2020.05.01.20087965. Available at: https://www.medrxiv.org/content/10.1101/2020.05.01.20087965 v3

Dimasi, D. *et al.* (2011) 'Ethnic and Mouse Strain Differences in Central Corneal Thickness and Association with Pigmentation Phenotype'. Available at: https://www.ncbi.nlm.nih.gov/pmc/articles/PMC3154201/

Do the Khoisan in Africa have Asian DNA? Considering they have an Asian phenotype? (no date) *Quora.* Available at: https://www.quora.com/Do-the-Khoisan-in-Africa-have-Asian-DNA-Considering-they-have-an-Asian-phenotype (Accessed: 2 July 2024).

Dupuis, M.L. *et al.* (2021) 'The role of vitamin D in autoimmune diseases: could sex make the difference?', *Biology of Sex Differences*, 12(1), p. 12. Available at: https://www.ncbi.nlm.nih.gov/pmc/articles/PMC7802252/

Fedorow, H. and Double, K.L. (2005) *Melanin - an overview ScienceDirect Topics*. Available at: https://www.sciencedirect.com/topics/neuroscience/melanin (Accessed: 4 August 2024).

Figure 1: Global map of skin pigmentation levels. This map, based on the... (no date) *ResearchGate*. Available at: https://www.researchgate.net/figure/Global-map-of-skin-pigmentation-levelsThis-map-based-on-the-work-of-the-geographer-R_fig5_8209215 (Accessed: 29 June 2024).

Jablonski, N.G. and Chaplin, G. (2017) 'The colours of humanity: the evolution of pigmentation in the human lineage', *Philosophical Transactions of the Royal Society B: Biological Sciences*, 372(1724), p. 20160349. Available at: https://www.ncbi.nlm.nih.gov/pmc/articles/PMC5444068/

Kaarthikeyan, G. (2021) 'Correlation of Skin Colour and Gingival Pigmentation Among Middle Aged Women In Chennai A Hospital Based Analysis', *International Journal of Dentistry and Oral Science*, pp. 1789–1792. Available at: https://www.academia.edu/58693323/Correlation_Of_Skin_Colour_and_Gingival_Pigmentation_Among_Middle_Aged_Women_In_Chennai_A_Hospital_Based_Analysis_Research_Article

'Khoisan' (2024) *Wikipedia*. Available at: https://en.wikipedia.org/w/index.php?title=Khoisan&oldid=1223800913.

Kohlmeier, M. (2020) 'Avoidance of vitamin D deficiency to slow the COVID-19 pandemic', *BMJ Nutrition, Prevention & Health*, 3(1), p. 67. Available at: https://nutrition.bmj.com/content/early/2020/05/20/bmjnph-2020-000096

Lin, L.-Y. *et al.* (2022) 'The association between vitamin D status and COVID-19 in England: A cohort study using UK Biobank', *PLOS ONE*, 17(6), p. e0269064. Available at: https://pubmed.ncbi.nlm.nih.gov/35666716/

Liu, J., Bitsue, H.K. and Yang, Z. (2024) 'Skin colour: A window into human phenotypic evolution and environmental adaptation', *Molecular Ecology*, 33(12), p. e17369. Available at: https://pubmed.ncbi.nlm.nih.gov/38713101/

Loomis, W.F. (1967) 'Skin-Pigment Regulation of Vitamin-D Biosynthesis in Man', *Science*, 157(3788), pp. 501–506. Available at: https://pubmed.ncbi.nlm.nih.gov/6028915/

Malaguarnera, L. (2020) 'Vitamin D3 as Potential Treatment Adjuncts for COVID-19', *Nutrients*, 12(11), p. 3512. Available at: https://www.ncbi.nlm.nih.gov/pmc/articles/PMC7697253/

Manager, M.M.-M.S.L. (2022) '7 very common skin diseases and their relationship with genetics', *Genes Matter*, 23 June. Available at: https://www.veritasint.com/blog/en/7-very-common-skin-diseases-and-their-relationship-with-genetics/ (Accessed: 4 July 2024).

MC1R gene: MedlinePlus Genetics (no date). Available at: https://medlineplus.gov/genetics/gene/mc1r/ (Accessed: 22 June 2024).

Fedorow, H. and Double, K.L. (2005) *Melanin - an overview | ScienceDirect Topics.* Available at: https://www.sciencedirect.com/topics/neuroscience/melanin (Accessed: 4 August 2024).

Intersectional Self - FYS 101 - Research Guides at Syracuse University Libraries (no date). Available at: https://researchguides.library.syr.edu/fys101/intersectionality (Accessed: 3 August 2024).

Is eye color determined by genetics?: MedlinePlus Genetics (no date). Available at: https://medlineplus.gov/genetics/understanding/traits/eyecolor/ (Accessed: 4 August 2024).

"Is This Because I'm Black?": A Story of Racial Discrimination | TLNT (no date). Available at: https://www.tlnt.com/articles/is-this-because-im-black-a-story-of-racial-discrimination (Accessed: 1 August 2024).

Mendoza-Denton, R. (2011) *Racism Against Whites: What's the Problem? | Psychology Today United Kingdom.* Available at: https://www.psychologytoday.com/gb/blog/are-we-born-racist/201103/racism-against-whites-whats-the-problem (Accessed: 4 August 2024).

Pavan, M.E., Lopez, N.I. and Pettinari, M.J. (2020) *Simplified pathways of tyrosine-derived melanin synthesis showing... | Download Scientific Diagram.* Available at: https://www.researchgate.net/figure/Simplified-pathways-of-tyrosine-derived-melanin-synthesis-showing-enzymatic-steps-subject_fig2_337820571 (Accessed: 4 August 2024).

Pavid, K. (2016) *Earliest evidence of modern humans breeding with Neanderthals | Natural History Museum*. Available at: https://www.nhm.ac.uk/discover/news/2016/february/earliest-evidence-humans-breeding-neanderthals.html?gad_source=1&gclid=EAIaIQobChMI_sz65dvYhwMVHZxQBh3PfRJwEAAYASAAEgJDYvD_BwE (Accessed: 3 August 2024).

Racism in Classic Pieces of Nordic Children's Literature (no date). Available at: https://nordics.info/show/artikel/racism-in-nordic-childrens-literature (Accessed: 4 August 2024).

Reformed skinhead endures agony to remove tattoos (no date). Available at: https://www.nbcnews.com/id/wbna45095048 (Accessed: 1 August 2024).

Section One- What Causes Tanning Of The Skin? | Utah County Health Department (no date). Available at: https://health.utahcounty.gov/online-tanning-certification-course/what-causes-tanning-of-the-skin/ (Accessed: 10 August 2024).

SIRT7 gene knockout using CRISPR/Cas9 system enhances melanin production in the melanoma cells - PubMed (no date). Available at: https://pubmed.ncbi.nlm.nih.gov/34303808/ (Accessed: 4 August 2024).

Skin cancer - tanning - Better Health Channel (no date). Available at: https://www.betterhealth.vic.gov.au/health/conditionsandtreatments/skin-cancer-tanning (Accessed: 10 August 2024).

TYR gene: MedlinePlus Genetics (no date). Available at: https://medlineplus.gov/genetics/gene/tyr/ (Accessed: 4 August 2024).

Vitamin D | International Osteoporosis Foundation (no date). Available at: https://www.osteoporosis.foundation/health-professionals/prevention/nutrition/vitamin-d (Accessed: 4 August 2024).

Scaria, S.S.& V. (2024) 'How genetics is revealing skin colour biology is more than skin-deep', *The Hindu*, 7 April. Available at: https://www.thehindu.com/sci-tech/science/skin-colour-diversity-genes-melanin-research/article68038937.ece (Accessed: 22 June 2024).

SIRT7 gene knockout using CRISPR/Cas9 system enhances melanin production in the melanoma cells. Available at:

https://pubmed.ncbi.nlm.nih.gov/34303808/

Sizar, O. *et al.* (2024) 'Vitamin D Deficiency', in *StatPearls*. Treasure Island (FL): StatPearls Publishing. Available at: http://www.ncbi.nlm.nih.gov/books/NBK532266/ (Accessed: 29 June 2024).

Skin diseases and conditions in darker skin tones (no date). Available at: https://www.aad.org/public/darker-skin/diseases (Accessed: 4 July 2024).

Thawabteh, A.M. *et al.* (2023) 'Skin Pigmentation Types, Causes and Treatment—A Review', *Molecules*, 28(12), p. 4839. Available at: https://www.ncbi.nlm.nih.gov/pmc/articles/PMC10304091/

Thompson, M. (2015) *How Birds Make Colorful Feathers | Bird Academy • The Cornell Lab*. Available at: https://academy.allaboutbirds.org/how-birds-make-colorful-feathers/ (Accessed: 1 July 2024).

Tishkoff Lab / Sarah Tishkoff, Ph.D. (no date). Available at: https://www.med.upenn.edu/tishkoff/Lab/Tishkoff/Tishkoff.html (Accessed: 6 July 2024).

Fedorow, H. and Double, K.L. (2005) *Melanin - an overview | ScienceDirect Topics.* Available at: https://www.sciencedirect.com/topics/neuroscience/melanin (Accessed: 4 August 2024).

Intersectional Self - FYS 101 - Research Guides at Syracuse University Libraries (no date). Available at: https://researchguides.library.syr.edu/fys101/intersectionality (Accessed: 3 August 2024).

Is eye color determined by genetics?: MedlinePlus Genetics (no date). Available at: https://medlineplus.gov/genetics/understanding/traits/eyecolor/ (Accessed: 4 August 2024).

"Is This Because I'm Black?": A Story of Racial Discrimination | TLNT (no date). Available at: https://www.tlnt.com/articles/is-this-because-im-black-a-story-of-racial-discrimination (Accessed: 1 August 2024).

Mendoza-Denton, R. (2011) *Racism Against Whites: What's the Problem? | Psychology Today United Kingdom.* Available at: https://www.psychologytoday.com/gb/blog/are-we-born-racist/201103/racism-against-whites-whats-the-problem (Accessed: 4 August 2024).

Pavan, M.E., Lopez, N.I. and Pettinari, M.J. (2020) *Simplified pathways of tyrosine-derived melanin synthesis showing... | Download Scientific Diagram.* Available at: https://www.researchgate.net/figure/Simplified-pathways-of-tyrosine-derived-melanin-synthesis-showing-enzymatic-steps-subject_fig2_337820571 (Accessed: 4 August 2024).

Pavid, K. (2016) *Earliest evidence of modern humans breeding with Neanderthals | Natural History Museum.* Available at:

https://www.nhm.ac.uk/discover/news/2016/february/earliest-evidence-humans-breeding-neanderthals.html?gad_source=1&gclid=EAIaIQobChMI_sz65d vYhwMVHZxQBh3PfRJwEAAYASAAEgJDYvD_BwE (Accessed: 3 August 2024).

Racism in Classic Pieces of Nordic Children's Literature (no date). Available at: https://nordics.info/show/artikel/racism-in-nordic-childrens-literature (Accessed: 4 August 2024).

Reformed skinhead endures agony to remove tattoos (no date). Available at: https://www.nbcnews.com/id/wbna45095048 (Accessed: 1 August 2024).

Section One- What Causes Tanning Of The Skin? | Utah County Health Department (no date). Available at: https://health.utahcounty.gov/online-tanning-certification-course/what-causes-tanning-of-the-skin/ (Accessed: 10 August 2024).

SIRT7 gene knockout using CRISPR/Cas9 system enhances melanin production in the melanoma cells - PubMed (no date). Available at: https://pubmed.ncbi.nlm.nih.gov/34303808/ (Accessed: 4 August 2024).

Skin cancer - tanning - Better Health Channel (no date). Available at: https://www.betterhealth.vic.gov.au/health/conditionsandtreatments/skin-cancer-tanning (Accessed: 10 August 2024).

TYR gene: MedlinePlus Genetics (no date). Available at: https://medlineplus.gov/genetics/gene/tyr/ (Accessed: 4 August 2024).

Vitamin D | International Osteoporosis Foundation (no date). Available at: https://www.osteoporosis.foundation/health-professionals/prevention/nutrition/vitamin-d (Accessed: 4 August 2024).

Vitamin D Deficiency & Skin Type: What You Need to Know | Cue (2023). Available at: https://cuehealth.com/blog/wellness/2023/07/06/vitamin-d-deficiency-skin-type-what-you-need-to-know (Accessed: 20 June 2024).

VITAMIN D: Overview, Uses, Side Effects, Precautions, Interactions, Dosing and Reviews (no date). Available at: https://www.webmd.com/vitamins/ai/ingredientmono-929/vitamin-d (Accessed: 21 June 2024).

Vitamin D2 vs. D3: What's the Difference? (2018) *Healthline*. Available at: https://www.healthline.com/nutrition/vitamin-d2-vs-d3 (Accessed: 21 June 2024).

Watson, S., King, L.M., and PhD (no date) *Vitamin D Deficiency: Symptoms, Causes, and Health Risks*, *WebMD*. Available at: https://www.webmd.com/diet/vitamin-d-deficiency (Accessed: 3 July 2024).

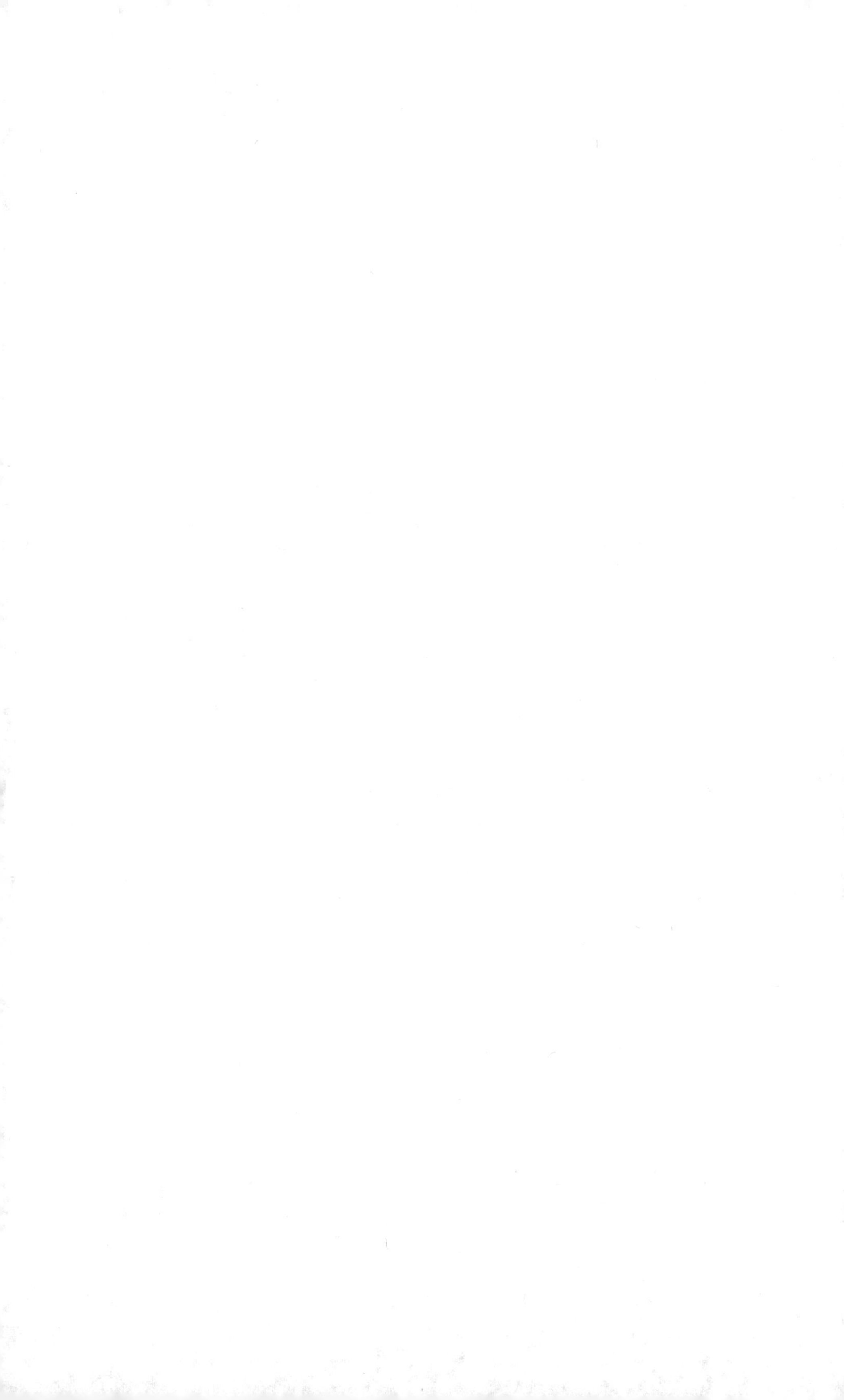

www.ingramcontent.com/pod-product-compliance
Lightning Source LLC
Chambersburg PA
CBHW071023250726

48653CB00005B/1684